ULTRASOUND IN HIGH-RISK OBSTETRICS

CURRENT CONCEPTS IN OBSTETRICS AND GYNECOLOGY

FREDERICK P. ZUSPAN, M.D., *Editor*

Department of Obstetrics and Gynecology
Professor and Chairman
The Ohio State University College of Medicine
    and
Obstetrician-Gynecologist-in-Chief
University Hospitals
Columbus, Ohio

ULTRASOUND
IN HIGH-RISK
OBSTETRICS

RUDY E. SABBAGHA, M.D.

Associate Professor of Obstetrics and Gynecology
Director of Diagnostic Ultrasound
Northwestern University Medical School
Prentice Women's Hospital
Chicago, Illinois

LEA & FEBIGER • 1979 • PHILADELPHIA

Library of Congress Cataloging in Publication Data

Sabbagha, Rudy E
  Ultrasound in high-risk obstetrics.

  (Current concepts in obstetrics and gynecology)
  Includes index.
  1. Ultrasonics in obstetrics. 2. Pregnancy, Complications of—Diagnosis. I. Title. [DNLM: 1. Fetal
diseases—Diagnosis. 2. Obstetrics. 3. Pregnancy
complications—Diagnosis. 4. Ultrasonics—Diagnostic
use. WQ240 S114u]
RG527.5.U48S22   618.3'07'54   79-15161
ISBN 0-8121-0676-8

Published in Great Britain by Henry Kimpton Publishers, London

PRINTED IN THE UNITED STATES OF AMERICA

Print number: 3   2   1

To
My wife Asma,
son Elias,
and
daughter Randa

FOREWORD

This monograph on ultrasound in perinatology by one of the early investigators in the field, Dr. Rudy Sabbagha, is a most welcome addition to the armamentarium of physicians who care for pregnant women. More importantly, Dr. Sabbagha brings to the reader the point of view of the obstetrician-gynecologist who specializes in maternal-fetal medicine.

As one gets older, one tends to ruminate about issues of the past and present. One of the issues of our society is the privilege of being wellborn. Fortunately, we are now in the era of what I term "scientific obstetrics" that has gradually emerged over the past eight to ten years. A major advance for the obstetrician during this period has been ultrasound. He can now instantly date pregnancies and diagnose many conditions such as placenta previa, multiple gestations, and fetal death. The management of these conditions is now seen in a different context since the diagnosis is certain, and one is no longer forced to play the waiting game in the management of the patient.

Medicine should thank the specialty of obstetrics since its practitioners were the first to embrace the science of ultrasound. Thanks to many obstetricians and their tenacity with early ultrasound machines, the science has now advanced, and other specialties have begun to use ultrasound with great frequency. One of the first five-shades-of-gray ultrasound machines was made by Zenith Radio Corporation in 1968 and tested when I was at the Chicago Lying-In Hospital. It was a gigantic piece of equipment that required technical expertise to maintain. This prototype was never again reproduced since a corporate decision dictated that Zenith abandon biomedical engineering. Since then, major advances in ultrasound include a shrinkage in equipment size and the advent of real-time ultrasound. Most importantly, the companies have made the equipment physician-proof, and there is little downtime. All of these advances mean better patient care and mechanisms by which we can better understand fetal physiology, which will result in healthier offspring and a stronger nation.

FREDERICK P. ZUSPAN, M.D.

PREFACE

High-risk obstetrics is a broad area encompassing not only maternal medical, surgical, and obstetric complications but also fetal medicine. Recent technologic advances have permitted the close monitoring of the biochemical and biophysical profiles of the fetus. Ultrasound is a new biophysical means of evaluating pregnancy, and because of its accuracy and noninvasive nature, the indications for its use throughout gestation have increased markedly.

The obstetrician at present is placed in a position of having to learn all about ultrasound—when to order the test and how to interpret the results. However, this is not all, for the introduction of the linear-array transducer producing real-time imaging has enthused many obstetricians to the point of actually purchasing the apparatus and learning the technique of scanning their own population of pregnant women.

Only a few years ago, in 1970, Professor Ian Donald, the father of obstetric sonar, wondered as he addressed the Royal College of Obstetricians and Gynecologists, why sonar was not yet widely utilized both in Britian and in the developed world. He stressed, even then, that he had been successfully using this remarkable tool for almost a decade.

The change in the attitude of obstetricians toward sonar may appear, on the surface, to be dramatic, but it really is long overdue and serves as another reminder of the historic fact: Change can only come with time.

The time for learning ultrasound is now. Dr. Zuspan, editor of the series, *Current Concepts in Obstetrics and Gynecology,* realizing the need for education in this area, asked me to present, in a concise way, the present-day applications of diagnostic ultrasound in high-risk pregnancy.

To give the reader an appreciation of the way in which ultrasound works and of its accuracy and reliability, the first two chapters deal with instrumentation and methodology.

The remaining four chapters contain descriptions and illustrations of the specific use of sonar in the antenatal detection of abnormal pregnancies. I am hopeful that in this way the efforts of all individuals participating in the care of pregnant women can be directed toward the fetus at risk, in an attempt to decrease its perinatal morbidity and mortality and to improve the quality of its life for many years to come.

Chicago, Illinois   RUDY E. SABBAGHA

ACKNOWLEDGMENTS

I wish to thank Ms. Patricia DeLung, Ms. Sally Fuller, and Ms. Merle Bent for their secretarial support. I am indebted to Ms. Debbie Cetera and Ms. Colleen Nelson for their outstanding assistance in putting the manuscript together. I would like to extend my gratitude to the technologists who have helped me plan my work schedule—Ms. Ingrid Kipper, Ms. Patricia Gannon, and Ms. Sharon DalCompo. My thanks also go to Scott Schlesser for reproducing the photographs in this text. Last but not least, I wish to thank Laurence E. Stempel, MD and Carl Weiner, MD for reviewing this manuscript and offering constructive criticism.

CONTENTS

1

INSTRUMENTATION

In the last few years, significant technologic advances in the field of ultrasonic instrumentation have resulted in: (1) improvement in the visualization of structures examined and, in turn, application of sonar to a wide range of clinical conditions; (2) simplification in the acquisition of scanning skills; and (3) shortening of the time allocated for completion of any given scan—an advantage that translates into utilization of the modality for a larger number of patients at reduced cost.

The principle of echography depends on the transmission of a pulsed sound beam through a particular area of the body and on the interpretation of the echo pattern produced from interfaces of tissues with different acoustic impedances or densities.

Transmission of Sound. Sound energy is formed when a piezoelectric crystal or transducer (Figs. 1–1 and 1–2) is excited by a pulsed electric current. The frequency of the sound beam emitted is related to the structure and diameter of the transducer. The frequency generally employed in the field of obstetrics and gynecology is 1.5 to 5 MHz (million vibrations/second). At this frequency, the intensity in tissues is of the order of 10 milliwatts/cm^2—energy levels that thus far do not appear to produce harmful effects in humans (see Chap. 5).

The depth of penetration of sound waves is inversely related to the frequency, i.e., the lower the frequency, the greater the depth. Thus, the use of low-frequency sound may appear advantageous for scanning structures situated more posteriorly in the field of examination. However, the resolution of echograms produced by transducers emitting low-frequency sound is poor. The wavelength of low-frequency sound is long, and resolution or distinction between two interfaces situated close to each other along the path of the beam (i.e., axially) is lost.

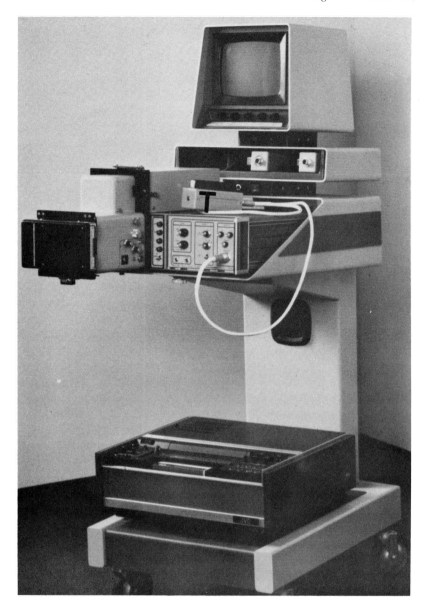

Figure 1–1.   *Real-time apparatus (ADR, Sy₂ model). A linear-array transducer (T) is used. Note: Transducer is attached to a flexible cord and can be easily angled to any position for display of the best obtainable image from the most appropriate plane. (Courtesy—Advanced Diagnostic Research [ADR] Corporation.)*

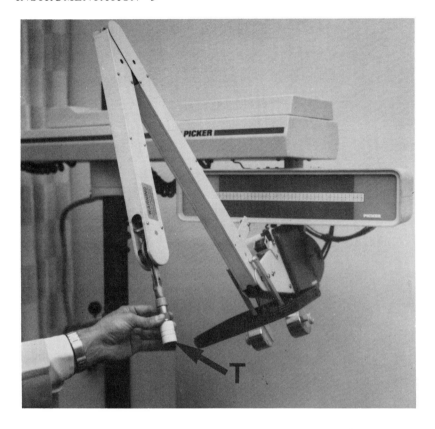

Figure 1–2. *A single transducer (T) is seen in transverse position and is angled for obtaining biparietal diameter (see text). (Courtesy—Picker Corporation.)*

Stated differently, axial resolution of echograms obtained by low-frequency sound (long wavelength) is poor.

Similarly, lateral resolution (recognition of echoes from interfaces perpendicular to the path of sound) is less than optimal when transducers emitting low-frequency sound are used because the sonic beam is both wide and divergent or not focused.

It is apparent, then, that total resolution of any ultrasonic system is substantially governed by both frequency and wavelength. Ideally, the transducer used should emit a nondivergent or focused beam in the zone of interest and produce the highest frequency that will penetrate to the desired depth.

Finally, the velocity at which sound traverses a particular area of the human body is determined by characteristics of the transmitting medium and is related to the product of frequency and wavelength. The average velocity of sound in soft tissue is universally accepted as 1540 meters/second (m/s).

Echoes. As previously mentioned, echoes are produced at the junction or interface of tissues of different acoustic impedances. These echoes, as in optics, return to the transducer only if the sound beam strikes the interface perpendicularly—otherwise they are reflected away from the transducer and are not recorded on the face of the cathode ray tube (crt) or television monitor. Experienced sonographers continually attempt to direct the sound beam to an angle perpendicular to structures examined. In this way, echoes from a greater number of interfaces are recovered, producing echograms of superior quality. In diagnostic ultrasound the transducer is pulsed (excited) at a rate of approximately 1000 times/s; thus, for the most part (99.9% of the time), it is receiving echoes and converting sound to electric energy (reverse piezoelectric effect).

Time-Gain Control (TGC). The signals reflected from posterior interfaces of the body are of low amplitude in comparison to more anterior echoes. The reason is attenuation of sound in distal areas secondary to reflection, absorption, and dissipation.

Thus, a TGC mechanism is incorporated in all sonar equipment and results in progressive amplification of echoes in relation to the depth of the interface. The curve of the TGC control knobs is shown in Figure 1–3.

In most sonar apparatus, overall gain may also be increased or decreased, i.e., the TGC curve can be elevated or lowered without altering its shape.

The different modes by which echoes are processed to a visually recognizable pattern are listed in Table 1–1 and are discussed separately.

A Mode (Amplitude Mode). In the A mode, echoes are deflected within the oscilloscope and appear as vertical spikes of the horizontal time-base sweep (Fig. 1–4). The amplitude (height of the spike) represents the strength of the echo and is measured in decibels (dB).

A-Mode Cephalometry. When the A mode is used to measure fetal biparietal diameter (BPD), three echoes are produced (Fig. 1–4). The

Figure 1–3. *Digital scan converter apparatus. Note progressive increase in the curve of the TGC knobs (arrow). (Courtesy—Picker Corporation.)* ⟶

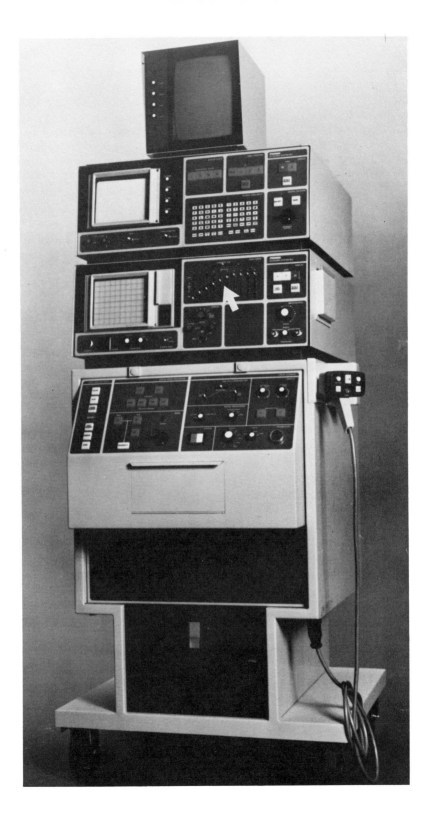

Table 1–1.   *Diagnostic Ultrasound Imaging Modalities*

Mode	Transducer	Scan	Dimension	Format
A (amplitude)	Single	Contact	Unidimensional	Oscilloscope
B (brightness)	Single	Contact	Two-dimensional	Oscilloscope
T-M (time-motion)	Single	Contact	Uni- or two-dimensional	Oscilloscope Television (TV)
Gray scale				
Amplitude modulation	Single	Contact	Two-dimensional	Oscilloscope
O–I Octosone	Multiple	Water Tank	Two-dimensional	Oscilloscope
Scan converter (analog, digital)	Single	Contact	Two-dimensional	Television (TV)
Real-time*	Multiple	Contact	Two-dimensional	Oscilloscope

*Linear array.

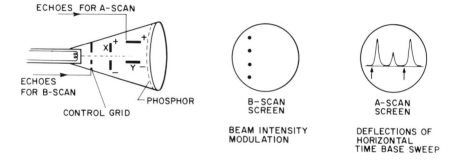

Figure 1–4.   *Echoes in B scan appear as bright dots of light; echoes in A scan appear as vertical deflections of horizontal time-base sweep. Arrows in A scan are pointing to the leading edges of the first and third echoes produced from the fetal head and represent an outer to inner (O–I) measurement of the BPD (see text).*

first is reflected from the outer aspect of the fetal head near the transducer. The second or small echo is returned from the interface between both cerebral hemispheres. The third echo represents the interface between the brain and distal skull table. As a result, the BPD obtained by the A mode is not a true anatomic dimension but one reflecting the distance from the outer to the inner (O–I) aspects of the fetal head (width of distal skull table and scalp is excluded); it is known

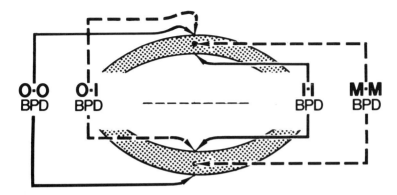

Figure 1–5. *BPD: biparietal diameter; O–O: BPD measured from outer points of cephalic contour; O–I: BPD measured from outer to inner aspect of cephalic contour (i.e., leading edge); M–M: BPD measured from midpoints of cephalic contour; I–I: BPD measured from inner aspect of cephalic contour. (From Hughey, M., Sabbagha, R.E.: Cephalometry by real-time imaging: A critical evaluation. Am. J. Obstet. Gynecol. 131:825, 1978.)*

as O–I BPD (Fig. 1–5).[1] In comparison, the anatomic BPD is the distance between the outer aspects of the fetal head and is known as O–O BPD (Fig. 1–5).[1]

The actual O–I BPD is measured by electronic calipers and represents the product of the time interval between the leading edges of the first and third echoes and the average velocity of ultrasound in soft tissue; for example, if this time interval is 0.000052 seconds and 1540 m/s is accepted as the average ultrasound tissue velocity, the BPD equals 0.000052 × 1540 or 8.0 cm.

Willocks et al. measured the width of the scalp and skull tables of fetuses of different gestational ages. They found that by using electronic calipers with an adjusted ultrasonic speed of 1600 m/s (instead of the conventional 1540 m/s) O–I BPDs may be automatically converted to O–O BPDs.[2] In this way, a sonar O–I BPD of 8 cm (at 1540 m/s) is inflated to an O–O BPD of 8.3 cm (8 × 1600/1540)—a difference of 3 mm.

In this ingenious method of transforming O–I to O–O BPDs, the increment is proportional to the progressive increase in the width of the distal skull table and scalp with advancing gestation. As an illustration, one should consider two fetuses with different O–I BPDs, namely, 6 cm and 8 cm. In adjusting these measurements to O–O BPDs, the respective increments are 2.3 mm and 3.5 mm—a difference of 1.2 mm.

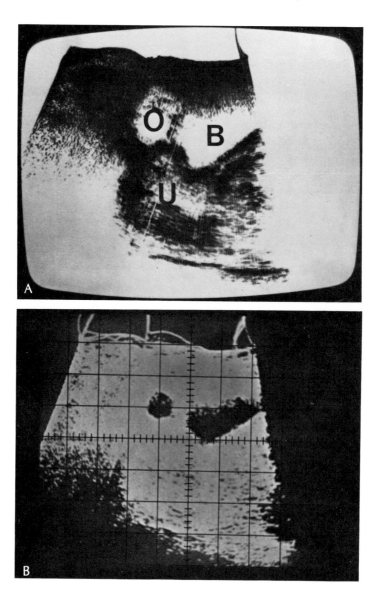

Figure 1-6.   A, *Shows uterus and ovarian cyst at high-gain settings used for gray-scale imaging. B = bladder; U = uterus; O = ovarian cyst. B, B-mode image of the same plane processed at similar gain settings. Note overwriting and loss of resolution—cyst is much smaller and uterus is not seen.*

B Mode (Brightness Mode). In the B mode echo signals strike and illuminate the phosphor of the oscilloscope screen and are visualized as bright dots of light along a vertical time sweep (Fig. 1–4). Movement of the ultrasound transducer over different areas within the field of examination coalesces these echoes or bright dots of light, displaying a two-dimensional image—a distinct technologic advance. However, in the B mode, echoes are not differentiated in relation to their amplitudes. Thus, macroscopic characteristics of tissues are not recorded. Additionally, increasing the gain or amplitude of return signals results in poor resolution because of overwriting or superimposition of echoes (Fig. 1–6).

Scanning. Introduction of B-mode two-dimensional sonar necessitated the development of scanning techniques. In essence, scanning represents an orderly search with the transducer probe along multiple longitudinal and transverse planes, and the mental transformation of the images produced to a three-dimensional scope.

The important scanning techniques are:

1. *The B scan.* In this method, the transducer probe is constantly moved in a position perpendicular to the surface examined.

2. *The compound-sector scan.* The transducer probe is rocked forward and backward through an angle of approximately 30° while simultaneously remaining perpendicular to the surface traversed.

3. *Nonpersistent image scanning (NPIS).* Continual rapid compound sector scanning is required to produce a nonpersistent image—one that instantly fades away if scanning is stopped. NPIS represents a dynamic method of scanning akin to real-time imaging, because movement of the transducer to different planes immediately results in the display of images from the new locations.[3]

Sonographers using NPIS are able to scan a wide anatomic field quickly and to locate the plane that best shows a particular normal or pathologic finding. Further, by using this method, the examiner can appreciate fetal motion as it occurs and be in a position to direct the transducer perpendicularly to structures of interest (e.g., BPD). Once the correct plane is located by NPIS, the image may be stored on an oscilloscope screen or on television (TV) format and examined; if it appears satisfactory, it is photographed and kept as a permanent record.[3]

NPIS is somewhat difficult to learn because it represents a combination of manual dexterity and rapid mental assimilation of images derived from multiple planes. Real-time imaging produced by a linear

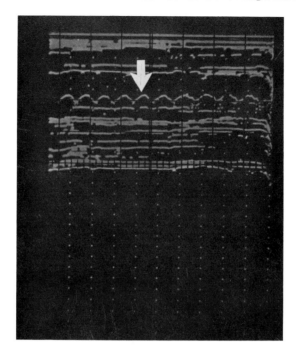

Figure 1–7. *Fetal heart motion as displayed on T-M mode (arrow).*

array of transducers has been introduced recently and is gaining widespread acceptance; it may be looked upon as an automatic and efficient means of producing NPIS with minimal operator skill. The application of real-time sonar to obstetrics is discussed elsewhere in this chapter.

Time-Motion (T-M) Mode. In the T-M presentation (used in echocardiography), the transducer is placed over the appropriate area, and echoes of moving structures are displayed as bright dots of light perpendicular to the horizontal time-base sweep. As a result, the motion of individual echoes is visualized and may be recorded on film or paper (Fig. 1–7).

Gray-Scale Sonography. Gray-scale sonography is based on technologic advances whereby echoes are recognized in relation to their amplitudes and the image produced is visually appreciated in eight shades of gray (Fig. 1–8). In this system, a much greater degree of echo information is retrieved, resulting in the display of gross characteristics of different tissues and enhancing diagnostic accuracy. Gray-scale echograms can be produced by a variety of electronic systems including:

1. *True-amplitude modulation.* In this gray-scale system, signal amplitude modulates the brilliance of the display oscilloscope. As a result, the range of spot brightness for each signal is increased, leading to gray-tone discrimination.[4]

2. *The U.I. octosone system.* Kossof et al. use a water tank covered by a polythene membrane.[5] The patient lies prone over the

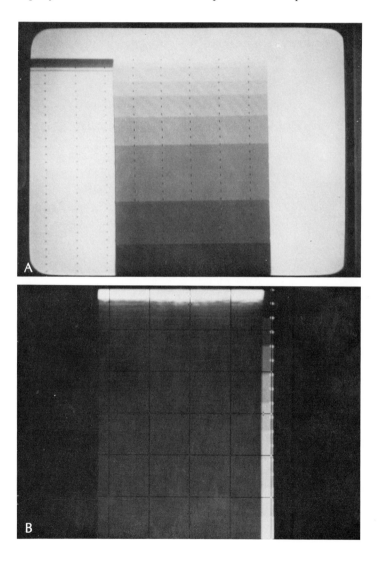

Figure 1–8. A, *Eight shades of gray as displayed by gray-scale apparatus.* B, *Eight shades of gray as displayed by real-time apparatus.*

membrane and is scanned by a number of transducers (placed in the water bath) oscillating mechanically every 2½ seconds. All echo signals above ground noise level are made to illuminate spots on a standard cathode ray oscilloscope screen. The image is recorded by continual open-shutter photography.

3. *Analog scan converter.* The most widely used forms of gray-scale apparatus are built with analog scan converters. Echo signals are directed to a target coated with silicon oxide and become uniformly distributed in accordance with their specific potential or amplitude. An electron beam is simultaneously used to transfer these signals to a television screen. Thus, all echoes, weak or strong, are represented and there is neither loss of information nor overwriting.

4. *Digital scan converter.* In this new system, a solid-state semiconductor device is used to store echoes in digital form, and digital circuitry rather than an electron beam is employed to convert echo signals into television format. The advantages of a digital scan converter are: (a) increase in the speed of writing; (b) elimination of the flicker apparent in analog systems; (c) consistent production of high-quality images because drift and focus problems are eliminated; and (d) future capability of utilizing computers to assign quantitative values to echo information—in the hope of defining digital patterns characteristic of different tissues or tumors.

Real-Time Imaging. Real-time is a mode of dynamic echography in which two-dimensional images are continually updated. Consequently, the motion of underlying structures is displayed as it occurs.

Real-time echography is particularly suitable for examination of the gravid uterus because, like NPIS, it allows the sonographer to scan a wide anatomic area with speed, appreciate fetal motion, and obtain accurate dimensions of fetal structures.

Three real-time scanners have been devised:

1. *Water-path scanner.* In this piece of equipment, the transducer is mounted on a cylindric arm placed in a water-filled tank and is rotated onto a parabolic reflecting mirror. A series of ultrasonic parallel beam lines is then projected through a coupling plastic window.

2. *Sector scanner.* In the sector scanner, single or multiple transducers are oscillated, and the image is displayed in sectors varying from 30° to 120°.

3. *Linear array scanner.* In this system, real-time imaging is produced by sequential firing of a linear array of transducers. Linear array scanners (see Fig. 1–1) are the most widely used form of real-time

equipment because of (a) small size; (b) low cost relative to gray-scale equipment; (c) portable capabilities; (d) ease of operation; (e) freely movable transducer readily directed to any desired angle; (f) possible use by obstetricians in an office situation and by sonographers in a hospital-based department; and (g) enhanced localization of the "appropriate plane" that best shows a normal or abnormal finding. The specific plane may then be scanned and displayed by a gray-scale unit for detailed analysis.

The limitations of this real-time system are related to the narrow field of visual display. For example, whereas careful examination of the pregnancy in the third trimester, using real-time, is possible, the whole fetus or placenta cannot be visualized at one time (see Chap. 5). Additionally, if vaginal bleeding occurs in gravidas close to term, the lower edge of the placenta in cases of borderline placenta previa may be difficult to localize by real-time imaging (see Chap. 6).

References

1. Hughey, M., and Sabbagha, R. E.: Cephalometry by real-time imaging: A critical evaluation. Am. J. Obstet. Gynecol., *131*:825, 1978.
2. Willocks, J., Donald, I., and Duggan, T.C.: Foetal cephalometry by ultrasound. J. Obstet. Gynaecol. Br. Commonw., *71*:11, 1964.
3. Sabbagha, R. E., and Turner, H. J.: Methodology of B-scan sonar cephalometry with electronic calipers and correlation with fetal birth weight. Obstet. Gynecol., *40*:74, 1972.
4. Railton, R., and Hall, A.J.: A simple approach to grey scale echography. Br. J. Radiol., *48*:921, 1975.
5. Kossof, G. et al.: Octoson: A new rapid multitransducer general purposes water-coupling echoscope. Excerpta Med. Internat. Cong. Series *No. 363*:90, 1975.

2

METHODOLOGY

Appreciation of the applicability and benefits of diagnostic ultrasound depends on knowledge of (1) the methodology used to obtain certain fetal dimensions and (2) the precision with which such measurements as fetal crown-rump length (CRL), biparietal diameter (BPD), and abdominal circumference (AC) relate to evaluation of fetal status.

This chapter describes some of the important sonar methods used in obstetrics. Moreover, the rationale behind standardization of cephalometry in relation to gestational age is presented.

Fetal Crown-Rump Length (CRL)

Robinson was the first to describe the method of localizing the longitudinal axis of the fetus in the first trimester of pregnancy for the purpose of obtaining a CRL measurement.[1] In his method, the fetal lie is localized by rapid scanning of the gestational sac along multiple parallel longitudinal planes. Subsequently, an echogram is obtained from the plane joining both fetal poles (Figs. 2–1 and 2–2).

Robinson's methodology may be time consuming because in the early part of gestation fetuses exhibit continual motion within the gestational sac. Real-time imaging (see Chap. 1) has simplified the procedure of obtaining fetal CRL measurements. The sonographer using a real-time scanner appreciates fetal motion and can easily tilt the transducer (connected only to a cord, Chap. 1) to the angle most

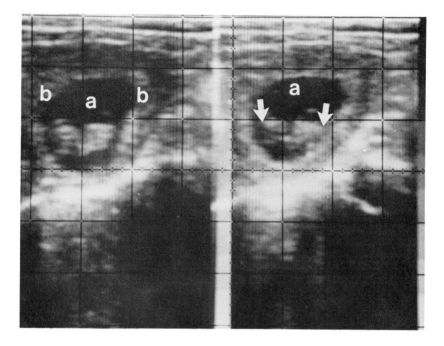

Figure 2–1. *Longitudinal scan of early pregnancy by real-time. Two pictures of the pregnancy are taken on one Polaroid film. Both gestational sacs show the crown-rump length (CRL) of the fetus. Arrows show limits of crown and rump; b = boundary of gestational sac; a = amniotic fluid.*

optimal for visualization of the correct plane featuring the CRL. The reproducibility of sonar measurements of the fetal CRL is ±1.2 millimeters in 95% of the population.[2]

Biparietal Diameter (BPD)

B–A Mode. Following the development of two-dimensional B-mode sonography, Campbell devised a method for measuring the fetal BPD, one which combines the B and A modes. First, by using NPIS, he localized the longitudinal axis of the fetus and then determined the extent of lateral flexion of the head (extent to which the fetus adjusts to the angle of pelvic inclination—normally 45°–55°) (Fig. 2–3). Second,

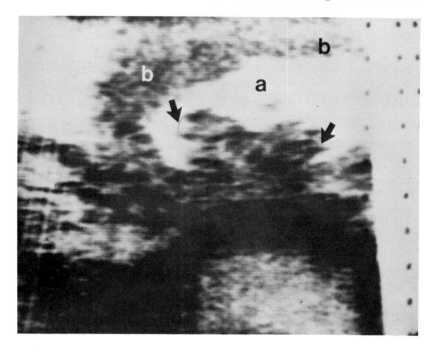

Figure 2–2.   *Gray-scale image of gestational sac and fetus. Arrows indicate limits of the fetal crown and rump; b = boundary of gestational sac; a = amniotic fluid.*

he moved the transducer to the transverse position (see Chap. 1, Fig. 1–2) and upon visualizing the correct BPD plane, he processed the echo signals to the A mode. It should be appreciated that if the fetal head is in an occiput anterior or posterior position the BPD cannot be obtained because it is technically difficult to angle the transducer perpendicular to the midline echo.

Electronic calipers were used to measure the distance between the leading edges of the cephalic echos (see Chap. 1). However, a read-out of an O–O BPD was obtained because calipers were calibrated to an ultrasound tissue velocity of 1600 m/s (see Chap. 1).

B Mode. Sabbagha et al. subsequently showed that the BPD plane can be localized by NPIS and immediately stored on the screen.[3] In this method, echoes from the skull tables were clearly visualized as bright dots of light (Fig. 2–4). Electronic calipers placed outside these echoes, however, still produced a digital read-out of an O–I BPD because the image of the distal skull table is extremely thin (Fig. 2–5).

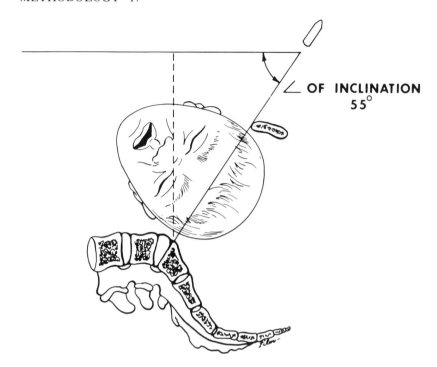

Figure 2–3. *The fetal head is laterally flexed as it adjusts to the angle of pelvic inclination.*

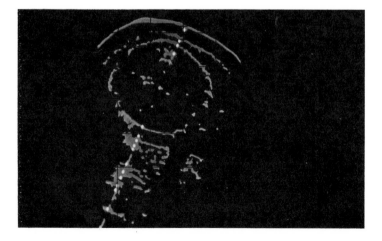

Figure 2–4. *Fetal cephalic contour obtained by B mode. Note bright dots of light over skull tables marking the points to be used for measuring the biparietal diameter.*

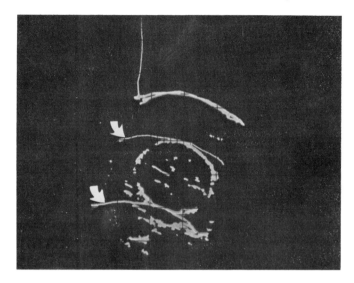

Figure 2–5. *Electronic calipers (arrows) are seen embracing the thin skull table echoes produced by B mode. The caliper read-out represents the outer to the inner (O–I) aspects of the biparietal diameter or O–I BPD.*

Table 2–1. *Factors Related to Reproducibility of Cephalometry*

Operator skill
Use of nonpersistent or real-time imaging
Symmetry of skull tables
Presence of midline echo
Cephalic points used to measure the biparietal diameter
Width of skull tables (related to gain)

BPD Charts. Since the advent of gray-scale and real-time imaging, the use of B mode for cephalometry has declined sharply. However, all reliable charts relating BPD to fetal age and growth were derived by B-mode technology. To determine whether such charts could be used to interpret BPD data derived by other imaging modalities, an analysis was made of the important factors pertaining to the reproducibility of cephalometry (Table 2–1). Of particular concern was the increased width of skull echoes produced by real-time and gray-scale apparatus and attributed to the high-gain settings used in this equipment.

Hughey and Sabbagha controlled the width of BPD skull tables by varying the gain settings, and they defined the relationship between these two variables (Table 2–2).[4] Subsequently, a number of fetuses were examined by different types of equipment and a comparison of all BPDs was analyzed statistically.[4] Interestingly, the differences among all O–I BPDs, regardless of the scanning modality used, were not statistically significant if the width of each skull table shown on gray-scale or real-time photographs was within 3 to 5 mm (Fig. 2–6).[4]

Table 2–2. *Definition of Width of Each Skull Table in Relation to Gain*

Gain	Stored Cephalic Image
	Width of each skull table (mm)
High	6–10
Medium	3–5
Low	1–2

From Hughey, M., and Sabbagha, R.E.: Cephalometry by real-time imaging: A critical evaluation. Am. J. Obstet. Gynecol., *131*:825, 1978.

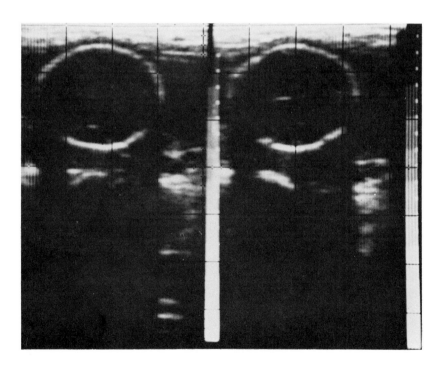

Figure 2–6. *Cephalic contour of fetal head obtained by real-time imaging. The width of skull tables (in relation to the centimeter marker scale) is about 3 mm.*

Table 2–3.   *Errors* in BPD Measurements Derived by Different Scanning Modalities*

Scanning techniques	BPD Measurement Error in mm (2SD)
B-A scan & NPIS[5]	$< \pm 1.0$
B-A scan & NPIS[6]	± 2.42
B-A scan & NPIS[6]	± 4.06
B-A scan & NPIS[7]	± 1.6
B-scan & NPIS[8]	± 1.0
Gray-Scale & NPIS[8]	± 1.6
Gray-Scale & stored imaging[8]	± 2.8
Real-Time[9]	± 1.54
Real-Time[4]†	± 0.8

* Errors noted represent ± 2SD.
† Width of each skull table is 3 to 5 mm.

Thus, to use the previously devised sonar charts (relating BPD to gestational age) O–I BPD measurements should be obtained from gray-scale and real-time photographs of the fetal head at medium-gain settings producing skull tables each only 3 to 5 mm wide.

Reproducibility of Cephalometry. In cephalometry, reproducibility is assessed by estimating the variance of several BPD readings obtained on one or more occasions, possibly by different technologists. Reproducibility of cephalometry is related to a number of factors listed in Table 2–1. A comparison of the reproducibility of BPD derived by different sonar modalities is shown in Table 2–3. It is apparent that variance in O–I BPD measurements (expressed as ±2SD) is smallest when real-time imaging is used and the width of each skull table is 3 to 5 mm.

Accuracy of Cephalometry. Cephalometric accuracy is gauged by correlating antenatal sonar BPDs with postnatal BPDs of fetuses delivered only by cesarean section—because of no cephalic molding.[9] Hughey and Sabbagha have shown that O–O BPDs measured from photographs derived by real-time imaging and in which each skull table is 3 to 5 mm wide correlate best with the anatomic BPDs of neonates delivered by cesarean section (Table 2–4).

Standardization of Cephalometry. In 1972, Sabbagha and Turner observed that various investigators reported different mean fetal BPD values in relation to each gestational week.[3] These differences were explained on the basis of possible inherent population variability or nonuniformity in the methodology of sonar cephalometry or both. At that time, sonographers were encouraged to use BPD data applicable to their respective laboratories.

As research in the field of fetal sonar cephalometry continued, the reasons for the apparent differences in charts relating BPD to gesta-

Table 2–4. *Biparietal Diameter: Sonar (Real-Time) vs. Neonatal Measurements*

BPD by Real-Time				Neontal BPD by Caliper Measurement after C-Section
High Gain Each Skull Table 6–10 mm Wide		Medium Gain Each Skull Table 3–5 mm Wide		
O–I	O–O	O–I	O–O	
8.0	9.0	8.1	8.50	8.5
8.5	9.2	8.4	8.85	8.8
8.3	9.2	8.5	8.95	8.9
8.6	9.3	8.9	9.25	9.2
9.2	9.8	9.0	9.50	9.7
9.3	10.0	9.3	9.70	9.8
8.8	9.8	8.9	9.40	9.2
9.0	9.7	9.1	9.60	9.5
9.1	9.8	9.3	9.75	9.7
9.4	10.0	9.3	9.70	9.7
9.8	10.6	9.6	9.9	10.0
9.6	10.5	9.7	10.0	9.9
9.6	10.4	9.6	10.1	10.0
9.6	10.2	9.8	10.1	10.2
9.5	10.3	9.6	10.0	10.0
9.7	10.6	9.9	10.2	10.0
9.8	10.6	10.0	10.35	10.3

BPD obtained either from the best of three photographs or from the mean of the best two of three photographs. O–O, out to out measurement of BPD. O–I, out to in measurement of BPD. Sonar M–M BPDs are almost identical to O–I BPDs and are not included. I–I BPDs differ significantly from neonatal BPDs and are excluded from this table. When each skull table is 3 to 5 mm wide (medium gain) the mean difference between sonar O–O BPDs and the true anatomic BPDs of neonates is not significantly different from zero. However, the mean difference between sonar O–I (leading edge) BPDs at either medium or high gain and BPDs of neonates is statistically significant (P<0.001). Similarly, the mean difference between sonar O–O BPDs at high gain and BPDs of neonates is statistically significant (P<0.001). O–I BPDs are smaller than actual BPDs of neonates by an average of 3.8 mm if medium gain is used and by an average of 4.5 mm if high gain is used.

From Hughey, M., and Sabbagha, R.E.: Cephalometry by real-time imaging: A critical evaluation. Am. J. Obstet. Gynecol., *131*:825, 1978.

tional age were clarified. It became apparent that the development of a standard BPD chart for universal use is not only possible but also highly desirable. A standard BPD chart derived from well-designed and well-executed studies would be reliable; further, it would lead to uniformity in the interpretation of BPD data pertaining to gestational age and to fetal growth.

Differences in BPD Charts. The reasons for the observed differences in BPD charts are:

1. *The use of different ultrasonic velocities in deriving the BPD.* As a result, some of the BPDs reported are O–I, while others are O–O measurements (because a velocity of 1600 m/s is used). The difference between O–I and O–O BPDs may be significant when an obstetrician is trying to assess feasibility of vaginal delivery in a breech presentation. In the latter case, an O–O BPD should be compared to pelvic size estimated clinically or radiologically.

2. *Lack of appreciation of the definition of gestational age.* In obstetrics, the duration of pregnancy is related to the first day of the last menstrual period and not to the approximate time of ovulation. However, many sonar charts relating BPD to gestational age are based on the assumed time of ovulation; their use leads to the incorrect underestimation of the length of pregnancy by 2 to 3 weeks.

3. *The use of storage B mode* rather than nonpersistent image scanning in obtaining BPDs from fetuses who are continually moving (see Chap. 1); the accuracy of such BPDs remains questionable.

4. *The placement of fetuses in highly specific gestational age categories in relation to single BPDs obtained in the third trimester of pregnancy.* For example, a BPD of 8.2 cm is reported to represent 32.3 weeks' gestation or a BPD of 9.0 cm is purported to denote maturity,[10] when the variation in gestational age for each of these readings is ±3 weeks (±2SD).[11] Such reports convey to the obstetrician an impression that cephalometry performed in the latter part of pregnancy is an extremely reliable method for prediction of fetal age and place him in a vulnerable position of false security.[12]

5. *Relating BPD data derived from pregnant women in geographic areas of high altitude* (approximately 6000 ft above sea level), where fetuses are known to be small, to gravidas living close to sea level.

6. *Measurement of BPD in relation to the scale on the face of the oscilloscope rather than in comparison to 1-cm markers (displayed on the screen) or electronic calipers.* In the former method BPD is artificially reduced in length because of parallax.

Table 2–5. *B-Scan Studies Relating Sonar BPD to Gestational Age*

Authors	Year	Number of Pregnancies	Number of BPDs*
Campbell & Newman[17]	1971	574	1029
Levi & Smets[18]	1973	1011	3032
Varma[19]	1973	100	1966
Sabbagha et al.[16]	1976	198	1032

* BPDs = biparietal diameters

In all studies BPDs were obtained by B scans or B–A scans from normal pregnant women with reliable dates who delivered normal neonates at term. None of the newborns were small for gestational age. Nonpersistent image scanning was utilized in all studies.

From Sabbagha, R.E., and Hughey, M.: Standardization of sonar cephalometry and gestational age. Obstet. Gynecol., *52*:405, 1978.

Similarity in BPDs. My colleagues and I compared the mean BPDs of black and caucasian fetuses between 20 to 40 weeks' gestation. A marked similarity was noted in both groups (Fig. 2–7).[13] Further, four well-executed B-scan studies relating BPD to gestational age (and utilizing similar methodology) were compared. In all, a mixed population of 1883 gravidas and 7059 BPD measurements were analyzed (Table 2–5).[12] The results showed that the mean differences in BPD values among the four groups and between each group and the composite mean (of all four studies) were not significantly different from zero.[12]

Standard Chart. The composite mean BPDs derived from the four studies cited above (Table 2–6) appear, logically, to be the values that should be used universally for prediction of gestational age. However, the range in the accuracy of defining the length of pregnancy by BPD depends on a variety of factors: (1) the interval during gestation at which cephalometry is performed: Single BPDs obtained prior to 26 to 28 weeks' gestation are more accurate than those measured later (Table 2–7); and (2) the number of BPD readings: Serial values obtained at approximately 20 and 30 weeks of pregnancy lead to an accurate prediction of gestational age by applying the principle of growth-adjusted sonar age (GASA) (see Chap. 3).

The composite mean BPD table or the first part of the GASA chart (see Chap. 3) may be used for predicting gestational age if a single BPD measurement is obtained early in the second trimester of pregnancy, e.g., prior to amniocentesis performed for genetic studies (see Chap. 5). However, for determining gestational age when serial cephalometry is performed, the GASA chart (statistically comparable to the composite BPD table) should be used. The reasons for this are discussed in Chapter 3. Similarly, when a single BPD is obtained in the third trimester of pregnancy, a chart comparable to the composite BPD table but also defining the probability estimates of fetal age should be used (see Chap. 3).

Table 2–6. *Mean Sonar BPDs Obtained from the 14th to 40th Weeks of Pregnancy Representing Four Different Studies with Uniform Methodology*

Week	Composite Mean	Sabbagha, et al.[13]	Campbell & Newman[17]	Varma[19]	Levi & Smets[18]
14	2.8	—	2.8	—	—
15	3.2	—	3.2	—	3.2
16	3.6	3.7	3.6	—	3.6
17	3.9	4.0	3.9	—	3.9
18	4.2	4.3	4.2	—	4.2
19	4.5	4.5	4.5	—	4.5
20	4.8	4.7	4.8	5.0	4.8
21	5.1	5.0	5.2	5.3	5.0
22	5.4	5.3	5.5	5.5	5.4
23	5.8	5.6	5.9	5.8	5.7
24	6.1	5.9	6.2	6.1	6.0
25	6.4	6.2	6.5	6.4	6.4
26	6.7	6.6	6.7	6.7	6.6
27	7.0	6.9	7.0	7.0	6.9
28	7.2	7.2	7.3	7.2	7.2
29	7.5	7.5	7.6	7.5	7.5
30	7.8	7.8	7.8	7.8	7.8
31	8.0	8.0	8.0	8.0	8.0
32	8.2	8.3	8.2	8.2	8.2
33	8.5	8.5	8.5	8.5	8.4
34	8.7	8.7	8.7	8.7	8.6
35	8.8	8.8	8.9	8.9	8.7
36	9.0	9.0	9.0	9.1	8.9
37	9.2	9.2	9.1	9.2	9.1
38	9.3	9.3	9.3	9.4	9.2
39	9.4	9.4	9.4	9.5	9.4
40	9.5	9.5	9.5	9.5	9.5

(1) BPDs obtained by B scans or B–A scans using nonpersistent image scanning. (2) All BPDs are measured from outer to inner aspects of fetal head (O–I BPD). (3) All BPDs shown are calculated from an ultrasonic tissue velocity of 1540 m/s. Original BPD data were not altered for Sabbagha et al. and Varma; it was reduced by a factor of 1540/1600 for Campbell and Newman, and increased by a factor of 1540/1529 for Levi and Smets.

From Sabbagha, R.E., and Hughey, M.: Standardization of sonar cephalometry and gestational age. Obstet. Gynecol., *52*:405, 1978.

Table 2–7. *Observed Variation in Gestational Age Predictions by BPDs Obtained During the Second and Third Trimesters of Pregnancy*

Week of Pregnancy BPD Is Obtained	Variation in Gestational Age by Days
16	±7*
17–26	±10–11†
27–28	±14*
29–40	±21*

* The reported variation in gestational age is applicable to 90% of fetuses.[13]
† The reported variation in gestational age is applicable to 95% of fetuses.[20]
    From Sabbagha, R.E., and Hughey, M.: Standardization of sonar cephalometry and gestational age. Obstet. Gynecol., *52*:405, 1978.

White vs Black Fetal BPD Growth Patterns

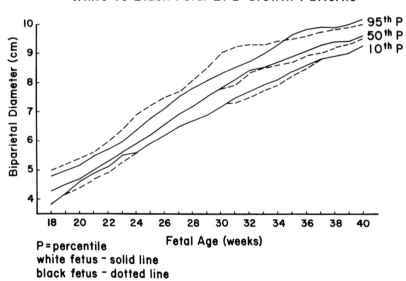

P = percentile
white fetus – solid line
black fetus – dotted line

Figure 2–7. *The mean BPD growth pattern of white and black fetuses is remarkably similar. (From Sabbagha, R. E., Barton, F. B., Barton, B. A.: Sonar biparietal diameter I. Analysis of percentile growth differences in two normal populations using same methodology. Am. J. Obstet. Gynecol. 126:479, 1976.)*

Abdominometry

Abdominometry is the term applied to the sonar measurement of the circumference of the fetal abdomen at the area of the liver where the umbilical vein is visualized (Fig. 2–7). These landmarks are chosen because they are easily reproducible and comparison of serial scans for assessment of fetal weight and growth is possible. Further, the liver is one of the organs whose size is noted to be small in the presence of intrauterine growth retardation.[14] Thus, in the presence of a small liver, abdominal girth is likely to be reduced. Similarly, there are data to indicate that when fetal nutrition is appropriate the circumference of the abdomen is large and may equal or exceed that of the head close to term.[15,16]

Methodology. In abdominometry, the sonographer should make sure that the scan is obtained at an angle perpendicular to the longitudinal axis of the fetus because an oblique section results in a circumference

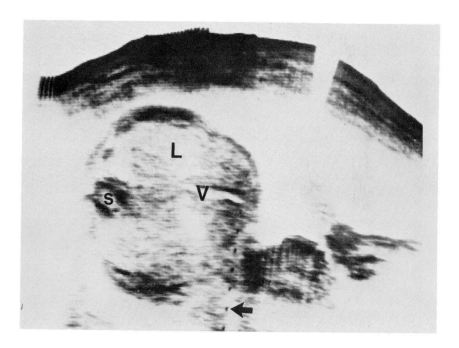

Figure 2–8. *Upper fetal abdomen displaying liver (L) and umbilical vein (V). This is the plane used for obtaining a circumference measurement of the fetal abdomen. Note centimeter scale (arrow head) and spine (S).*

measurement larger than the true anatomic dimension. Real-time imaging is particularly useful for this purpose because the fetal lie can be quickly identified and the plane perpendicular to the fetal axis located.

A variety of methods have been used to derive the abdominal circumference from a photograph of the fetus (featuring the liver and umbilical vein). The author prefers to use a digitizer (Fig. 2–8). The measurement is obtained as follows: First, the reduction in the scale of the photograph is determined by measuring the actual distance between two points along the centimeter scale projected on the Polaroid picture. Second, the outer perimeter of the fetal abdomen is transformed into digits (by the digitizer) and multiplied by a factor inversely proportional to the calculated reduction in the scale of the echogram.

As an illustration, if the distance between two points on the one-centimeter marker scale is reduced to 0.3 (actual centimeters) the circumference of the fetal abdomen derived by the digitizer (from the Polaroid photograph) is multiplied by a factor of 1.0/0.3. The error in the circumference measurement by this method is <2%.

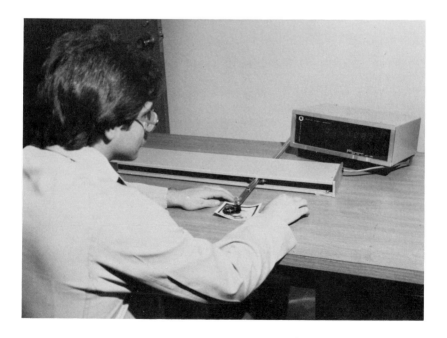

Figure 2–9. *Digitizer used to measure circumference of fetal abdomen.*

References

1. Robinson, H. P.: Sonar measurement of the fetal crown-rump length as a means of assessing maturity in the first trimester of pregnancy. Br. Med. J., *4*:28, 1973.
2. Robinson, H. P., and Fleming, J. E. E.: A critical evaluation of sonar crown-rump measurements. Br. J. Obstet. Gynaecol., *82*:702, 1975.
3. Sabbagha, R. E., and Turner, H. J.: Methodology of B-scan sonar cephalometry with electronic calipers and correlation with fetal birth weight. Obstet. Gynecol., *40*:74, 1972.
4. Hughey, M., and Sabbagha, R. E.: Cephalometry by real-time imaging: a critical evaluation. Am. J. Obstet. Gynecol., *131*:825, 1978.
5. Campbell, S.: Ultrasonic fetal cephalometry during the second trimester of pregnancy. J. Obstet. Gynaecol. Br. Commonw., *77*:12, 1970.
6. Davison, J. M., Lind, T., Farr, V., and Whittingham, T. A.: The limitations of ultrasonic fetal cephalometry. J. Obstet. Gynaecol. Br. Commonw., *80*:769, 1973.
7. Poll, V.: Precision of ultrasonic cephalometry. Br. J. Obstet. Gynaecol., *83*:217, 1976.
8. Sabbagha, R. E., Chilcote, W. S., Martin, A. O., and Grasse, D.: Reproducibility of ultrasonic cephalometry using B-scan and gray-scale imaging. Ultrasound Med., *3A*:663, 1977.
9. Copperberg, P. L., Chow, T., Kite, V., and Austin, S.: Biparietal diameter: A comparison of real-time and conventional B-scan techniques. J. Clin. Ultrasound, *4*:421, 1976.
10. Brown, R. E.: Ultrasonography: Basic Principles and Clinical Application. St. Louis: Warren H. Green, Inc., 1975.
11. Sabbagha, R. E. et al.: Sonar bipartietal diameter: II. Predictive of three fetal growth patterns leading to a closer assessment of gestational age and neonatal weight. Am. J. Obstet. Gynecol., *126*:435, 1976.
12. Sabbagha, R. E., and Hughey, M.: Standardization of sonar cephalometry and gestational age. Obstet. Gynecol., *52*:405, 1978.
13. Sabbagha, R. E., Barton, F. B., and Barton, B. A.: Sonar biparietal diameter: I. Analysis of percentile growth differences in two normal populations using same methodology. Am. J. Obstet. Gynecol., *126*:479, 1976.
14. Gruenwald, P.: Chronic fetal distress and placental insufficiency. Biol. Neonate, *5*:215, 1963.
15. Campbell, S., and Thoms, A.: Ultrasound measurement of fetal head to abdomen ratio in the assessment of growth retardation. Br. J. Obstet. Gynaecol., *84*:165, 1977.
16. Kurjak, A., and Breyer, B.: Estimation of fetal weight by ultrasonic abdominometry. Am. J. Obstet. Gynecol., *125*:962, 1976.
17. Campbell, S., and Newman, G. B.: Growth of the fetal biparietal diameter during normal pregnancy. J. Obstet. Gynaecol. Br. Commonw., *78*:513–519, 1971.
18. Levi, S., and Smets, P.: Intrauterine fetal growth studied by ultrasonic biparietal measurements. Acta Obstet. Gynecol. Scand., *52*:193, 1973.
19. Varma, T. R.: Prediction of delivery date by ultrasound cephalometry. J. Obstet. Gynaecol. Br. Commonw., *80*:316–319, 1973.
20. Sabbagha, R. E. et al.: Sonar BPD and fetal age: Definition of the relationship. Obstet. Gynecol., *43*:7, 1974.

3

FETAL AGE

In the prospective clinical management of high-risk gravidas, objective definition of the length of pregnancy is mandatory because gestational age is:

1. *Used as the basis for determining the expected date of delivery* (EDD).

2. *An important clinical index for determining the most optimal time for delivery.* In one study, perinatal mortality was shown to be four times greater in gravidas with uncertain dates than in those with established dates.[1]

3. *A guide for estimating whether the uterine fundus is either large or small for dates*—parameters that lead the obstetrician to rule out abnormalities such as polyhydramnios, oligohydramnios, intrauterine growth retardation, multiple pregnancy, molar pregnancy, and the possible presence of a pelvic mass.

4. *The x-coordinate of a multitude of graphs* (Table 3–1) dealing with the physical and biochemical profiles of the fetus. Interpretation

Table 3–1. *Parameters Reflecting Fetal Status In Relation To Gestational Age*

α-Fetoprotein (amniotic fluid)
Maternal estriol level
Human placental lactogen
Lecithin-sphingomyelin ratio
Growth of fetal biparietal diameter
Growth of fetal abdominal circumference
Estimation of fetal weight

of parameters shown in the graphs depends on the accuracy of assessment of fetal age. For example, a high α-fetoprotein value at 18 weeks of pregnancy falls within the normal range for a 16-week fetus.[2] Similarly, a specific estriol level in maternal urine or blood falling below two standard deviations in a pregnancy assumed to be 37 weeks in duration is considered normal if the correct fetal age is only 34 weeks.[3]

Fetal age is conventionally defined in relation to the first day of the last menstrual period (LMP). However, in 20% to 40% of pregnancies, the LMP is uncertain because of a variety of factors listed in Table 3–2.[4] Moreover, confirmation of gestational age is still necessary in high-risk obstetrics even when gravidas recall the LMP because in approximately 15% of such pregnancies, inaccurate menstrual dates are still reported.[5]

Sonography represents an objective, noninvasive biophysical means of defining gestational age with an accuracy superior to any other known methodology. By utilizing sonar, the length of pregnancy is ascertained from two measurements: fetal CRL and fetal BPD (see Chap. 2).

In formulating the relationship between fetal CRL and BPD measurements for each week of gestation, investigators were faced with the task of selecting gravidas with impeccable LMPs. The reason: difficulty was experienced in obtaining a large series of pregnant women in whom ovulation was timed. This meant that studies had to be performed on gravidas who fulfilled most, if not all, of the following criteria: (1) menstrual cycles were regular, occurring approximately every 26 to 30 days; (2) no oral contraceptives were used within at least 3 to 6 months prior to conception; and (3) delivery occurred spontaneously between 38 and 42 weeks' gestation and the fetus was considered to be at term and normal upon pediatric examination.

Table 3–2.   *Factors Relating To Uncertainty Of Menstrual Dates*

Inability to recall LMP*
Inaccurate reporting of LMP
Bleeding during pregnancy
Oligomenorrhea
Irregular periods
Use of oral contraceptives prior to pregnancy
Pregnancy in postpartum period

* LMP=first day of last menstrual period.

Robinson and Fleming defined the relationship between fetal CRL measurements obtained in the first trimester of pregnancy and fetal age.[6] They showed that fetal CRL can be used to predict gestational age with an accuracy of ±4.7 to ±2.7 days in 95% of gravidas depending on whether one or three CRL values were obtained, respectively. These data were verified by Drumm et al., who studied 40 gravidas in whom ovulation was established by basal body temperature records.[7]

Table 3–3. *Fetal Crown-Rump Length Measurements vs. Fetal Age*

Menstrual Maturity (weeks + days)	Corrected "Regressional Analysis" (cm) Mean Values	Menstrual Maturity (weeks + days)	Corrected "Regressional Analysis" (cm) Mean Values
6 + 2	0.55	10 + 2	3.32
6 + 3	0.61	10 + 3	3.46
6 + 4	0.68	10 + 4	3.60
6 + 5	0.75	10 + 5	3.74
6 + 6	0.81	10 + 6	3.89
7 + 0	0.89	11 + 0	4.04
7 + 1	0.96	11 + 1	4.19
7 + 2	1.04	11 + 2	4.35
7 + 3	1.12	11 + 3	4.51
7 + 4	1.20	11 + 4	4.67
7 + 5	1.29	11 + 5	4.83
7 + 6	1.38	11 + 6	5.00
8 + 0	1.47	12 + 0	5.17
8 + 1	1.57	12 + 1	5.34
8 + 2	1.66	12 + 2	5.52
8 + 3	1.76	12 + 3	5.70
8 + 4	1.87	12 + 4	5.88
8 + 5	1.97	12 + 5	6.06
8 + 6	2.08	12 + 6	6.25
9 + 0	2.19	13 + 0	6.43
9 + 1	2.31	13 + 1	6.63
9 + 2	2.42	13 + 2	6.82
9 + 3	2.54	13 + 3	7.02
9 + 4	2.67	13 + 4	7.22
9 + 5	2.79	13 + 5	7.42
9 + 6	2.92	13 + 6	7.63
10 + 0	3.05	14 + 0	7.83
10 + 1	3.18		

The mean crown-rump length and the corresponding gestational age are shown. The ±2 SD limits are ±4.7 days.[6]

The specific CRL values corresponding to weeks of gestation are shown in Table 3–3. The CRL may be used to define gestational age up to the thirteenth week of pregnancy; beyond this period the BPD is used.

Fetal BPD. The relationship between cephalometry and gestational age depends on whether single or serial BPD measurements are obtained.

Table 3–4. *BPD Percentile Ranges and Measurements for Both Black and White Fetuses*

Fetal age (week)	BPD percentiles							N
	5	10	25	50	75	80	95	
16	3.1	3.2	3.4	3.7	4.0	4.1	4.5	12
17	3.4	3.5	3.7	4.0	4.3	4.4	4.7	15
18	3.7	3.8	4.0	4.3	4.5	4.6	4.9	22
19	3.9	4.2	4.3	4.5	4.8	4.9	5.1	33
20	4.2	4.5	4.6	4.7	5.0	5.1	5.3	39
21	4.5	4.8	4.9	5.0	5.3	5.4	5.5	40
22	4.9	5.0	5.2	5.3	5.6	5.7	5.8	48
23	5.2	5.3	5.5	5.6	5.9	6.0	6.2	57
24	5.5	5.6	5.8	5.9	6.2	6.3	6.6	50
25	5.8	5.9	6.0	6.2	6.5	6.6	7.0	47
26	6.1	6.2	6.3	6.6	6.8	6.9	7.3	43
27	6.4	6.5	6.7	6.9	7.1	7.2	7.6	51
28	6.6	6.7	7.0	7.2	7.4	7.5	7.9	51
29	6.8	6.9	7.3	7.5	7.8	7.9	8.3	53
30	7.1	7.2	7.6	7.8	8.0	8.2	8.6	50
31	7.3	7.4	7.8	8.0	8.2	8.4	8.8	48
32	7.5	7.6	8.0	8.3	8.4	8.6	9.0	47
33	7.7	7.8	8.3	8.5	8.6	8.8	9.1	50
34	7.9	8.0	8.5	8.7	8.9	9.1	9.3	50
35	8.2	8.3	8.7	8.8	9.1	9.3	9.6	49
36	8.3	8.5	8.9	9.0	9.3	9.4	9.7	48
37	8.4	8.8	9.0	9.2	9.4	9.5	9.8	43
38	8.5	8.9	9.1	9.3	9.5	9.6	9.9	42
39	8.7	9.0	9.2	9.4	9.6	9.7	10.0	29
40	8.9	9.3	9.4	9.5	9.7	9.8	10.1	15

BPD percentile values from 16 to 40 weeks

From Sabbagha, R.E., et al.: Sonar biparietal diameter II. Predictive of three fetal growth patterns leading to a closer assessment of gestational age and neonatal weight. Am. J. Obstet. Gynecol., *126*:485, 1976.

Single BPDs. Sabbagha et al. have shown that a biologic variation in the length of the BPD exists for each week of gestation and that this variation increases as pregnancy advances (Fig. 3–1 and Table 3–4).

Prior to the 28th week of pregnancy, a single BPD is predictive of gestational age with an accuracy of ±11 days in 95% of the population. However, in the third trimester of pregnancy, the predictive accuracy of a single BPD is widened to ±3 weeks in 90% of the population (Table 3–5). If a single BPD is obtained prior to 28 weeks' gestation, the composite mean BPD table (detailed in Chap. 2) or the first part of the GASA chart (Table 3–6) should be used. However, if a single BPD is obtained in the third trimester of pregnancy, the correlation with gestational age for all fetuses (large and small BPDs) is too wide to be useful clinically. Nonetheless, the gestational age of a fetus with an average BPD may be expressed and reported with probability estimates within a 2- to 4-week range (Table 3–7).[8,9] In this way, the obstetrician is reminded that the length of pregnancy is not applicable to fetuses with large or small cephalic size.

Serial Cephalometry. Serial O–I BPD measurements (see Chap. 2), if obtained during defined intervals of pregnancy, are much more accurate indices of fetal age, namely, ±1–3 days (±2SD).[9] The reason is related to the finding that cephalic growth, under normal conditions, progresses within relatively narrow percentile limits. Specifically, Sabbagha et al. have shown that by mid pregnancy, BPDs in both the rhesus monkey and the human fetus can be classified into three subgroups: (1) large (BPD > the 75th percentile); (2) average (BPDs in the 25th to 75th percentiles) and (3) small (BPDs < the 25th percentile).[9,10] Thus, if the BPD subgroup of a given fetus is defined, the variation in gestational age is smaller and the length of the pregnancy can be assessed with greater accuracy. The method by which the BPD growth pattern is defined and gestational age assigned is termed growth-adjusted sonar age.[11]

Growth-Adjusted Sonar Age (GASA). As mentioned previously, the biologic variation in the BPD for each week of pregnancy (in the interval of 17–26 weeks) is ±11 days (2SD) (Figs. 3–1 and 3–2). For example, if the average length of pregnancy for a given fetus with a BPD of 5.7 cm is 23 weeks, gestational age can vary from 21+ to 24+ weeks (Table 3–5; Fig. 3–1). Careful analysis of Figures 3–1 and 3–2 shows that this variation is related to: (1) the younger fetus with a large BPD; and (2) the older fetus with a small BPD. Because the latter two fetuses cannot be differentiated from the first sonar BPD measurement, the mean gestational age of 23 weeks is assigned to all fetuses. In this way, however, the length of pregnancy is incorrectly advanced in the

Table 3–5.   *Fetal Age Percentile Values for BPDs from 3.5 to 9.5 cm*

BPD	Fetal age percentiles (week)*						
	5	10	25	50	75	80	95
3.5	17+	17	16+	16	16−	16−	15+
3.6	18	17+	17	16+	16	16	15+
3.7	19	18	18	17−	16	16	16
3.8	19	18+	18+	17	16+	16+	16
3.9	19+	19	18+	17+	17−	17−	16
4.0	19+	19	19−	18−	17	17−	16
4.1	19+	19	19−	18	17+	17+	16
4.2	20−	19+	19	18+	17+	17+	16+
4.3	20	20−	19+	19−	18−	18−	17−
4.4	20+	20	20−	19	18+	18	17
4.5	21−	20+	20	19+	19−	18	17+
4.6	21	21−	20+	20−	19	18+	18−
4.7	21+	21	21−	20	19+	19	18
4.8	21+	21	21	20+	20−	19+	18+
4.9	22−	21+	21+	21−	20	19+	19−
5.0	22	22	22−	21	20+	20−	19
5.1	22+	22	22−	21+	20+	20	19+
5.2	23−	22+	22	22−	21−	20+	20−
5.3	23	23−	22+	22−	21	21−	20
5.4	24−	23+	23−	22	21+	21+	20+
5.5	24	24−	23	22+	22−	21+	21−
5.6	24	24−	23+	23−	22	22−	21
5.7	24+	24	24−	23	22+	22+	21+
5.8	25−	24+	24	23+	23−	23−	21+
5.9	25	25−	24+	24−	23	23−	22−
6.0	25+	25	25−	24	23	23	22−
6.1	26−	25+	25	24+	23+	23+	22
6.2	26	26−	25+	25−	24−	23+	22+
6.3	26+	26	26−	25	24	24	23−
6.4	27−	26+	26	25+	24+	24+	23+
6.5	27+	27	26+	26−	25	25	24−
6.6	28−	27+	27−	26	25+	25+	24−
6.7	28	28−	27	26+	26−	26−	24

Table 3–5. *continued*

BPD	Fetal age percentiles (week)*						
	5	10	25	50	75	80	95
6.8	28+	28	27+	27−	26	26−	24+
6.9	29	28+	28−	27	26+	26+	25−
7.0	29+	29−	28	27+	27−	26+	25−
7.1	30	30−	28+	28−	27	27−	25+
7.2	31−	30−	29−	28−	27+	27	25+
7.3	31	30	29	28	28−	27+	26−
7.4	32−	31	29+	28+	28−	27+	26
7.5	32	32−	30−	29−	28+	28−	26+
7.6	33−	32	30	29	28+	28	27−
7.7	33	32	30+	30−	29−	28+	27
7.8	33	32+	31−	30	29−	29−	27+
7.9	33+	33	31+	30+	29	29	28−
8.0	34	33+	32	31−	29+	29+	28
8.1	34+	34	32+	31	30−	30−	28+
8.2	35	35−	33−	31+	30	30	29−
8.3	36−	35	33	32	31	30+	29
8.4	36	36−	33+	32+	31	31−	29
8.5	36+	36−	34−	33	31+	31	29+
8.6	36+	36−	34	33+	31+	31	29+
8.7	37−	36	35−	34	32−	31+	30−
8.8	37	36+	35+	34+	32	32−	30
8.9	38−	37	36	35+	33	32+	31
9.0	38+	37+	37−	36−	33+	33	32−
9.1	39−	38	37	36+	34	34	32+
9.2	39	39−	37+	36+	35	35	33
9.3	39+	39−	38−	37−	35	35	34−
9.4	40−	39	38	37	36−	35	34+
9.5	40	39+	38+	37+	36	35	35−

* + =1 to 3 days; − =1 to 3 days.

From Sabbagha, R.E., et al.: Sonar biparietal diameter II. Predictive of three fetal growth patterns leading to a closer assessment of gestational age and neonatal weight. Am. J. Obstet. Gynecol., *126*:485, 1976.

Table 3–6. *Chart for Assignment of Growth-Adjusted Sonar Age (GASA)*

	First sonar* (BPD vs fetal age percentile)		Fetal Age (week)	Second sonar (BPD percentile range)		
BPD	Range Large Fetus vs Small Fetus (week)	Average Fetus (age accepted temporarily)		Average Fetus (>25 to <75)	Large Fetus (75 to 95)	Small Fetus (5 to 25)
2.8	±1	14	29	7.4–7.7	7.8–8.3	6.8–7.3
3.2	±1	15	29+	7.5–7.8	7.9–8.4	6.9–7.4
3.5	±1	16	30–	7.6–7.8	7.9–8.5	7.0–7.5
3.6	±1.6	16+	30	7.7–7.9	8.0–8.6	7.1–7.6
3.7	±1.6	17–	30+	7.8–8.0	8.1–8.7	7.2–7.7
3.8	±1.6	17	31–	7.8–8.0	8.1–8.7	7.2–7.7
3.9	±1.6	17+	31	7.9–8.1	8.2–8.8	7.3–7.8
4.0	±1.6	18–	31+	8.0–8.2	8.3–8.9	7.4–7.9
4.1	±1.6	18	32–	8.0–8.2	8.3–8.9	7.4–7.9
4.2	±1.6	18+	32	8.1–8.3	8.4–9.0	7.5–8.0
4.3	±1.6	19–	32+	8.2–8.4	8.5–9.0	7.6–8.1
4.4	±1.6	19	33–	8.3–8.4	8.5–9.1	7.6–8.2
4.5	±1.6	19+	33	8.4–8.5	8.6–9.1	7.7–8.3
4.6	±1.6	20–	33+	8.5–8.6	8.7–9.2	7.8–8.4
4.7	±1.6	20	34–	8.5–8.7	8.8–9.2	7.8–8.4
4.8	±1.6	20+	34	8.6–8.8	8.9–9.3	7.9–8.5

BPD	Variation	Weeks			
4.9	±1.6	21−		8.0–8.6	
5.0	±1.6	21		8.1–8.6	
5.1	±1.6	21+		8.2–8.7	
5.2	±1.6	22−		8.2–8.8	
5.3	±1.6	22−		8.2–8.8	
5.4	±1.6	22		8.3–8.9	
5.5	±1.6	22+		8.4–9.0	
5.6	±1.6	23−		8.5–9.1	
5.7	±1.6	23		8.7–9.2	
5.8	±1.6	23+		8.9–9.4	
5.9	±1.6	24−			
6.0	±1.6	24			
6.1	±1.6	24+			
6.2	±1.6	25−			
6.3	±1.6	25			
6.4	±1.6	25+			
6.5	±1.6	26−			
6.6	±1.6	26			
7.5	±3	29−			
8.5	±3	33			
9.5	±3	37+			

Weeks	Range	Range
34+	8.7–8.9	9.0–9.4
35−	8.7–8.9	9.0–9.5
35	8.8–9.0	9.1–9.6
35+	8.9–9.0	9.2–9.6
36−	8.9–9.1	9.3–9.6
36	9.0–9.2	9.3–9.7
37	9.1–9.3	9.4–9.8
38	9.2–9.4	9.5–9.9
39	9.3–9.5	9.6–10.0
40	9.5–9.6	9.7–10.1

BPD measured from outer to inner aspects of fetal head; + = plus 1 to 3 days; − = minus 1 to 3 days.

* First sonar is done prior to 26 weeks because of small variation in fetal age of ± 11 days. Second sonar: (1) Must be done between 30 to 33 weeks because of maximal variation in fetal BPD size in this interval and prior to onset of IUGR in most cases. (2) Must be done at least 6 weeks after first BPD.

From Sabbagha, R.E., Hughey, M., and Depp, R.: Growth adjusted sonographic age: A simplified method. Obstet. Gynecol., *51*:384, 1978.

Table 3–7. *Range of Gestational Age in Fetuses With Average or Close to Average Cephalic Size in Relation to Single BPDs Obtained After 26 Weeks' Gestation*

BPD	Range in Gestational Age (weeks)*
6.7	25–27
6.8	26–28
6.9	26–28
7.0	26–29
7.1	26–29
7.2	26–29
7.3	27–30
7.4	27–30
7.5	28–31
7.6	28–31
7.7	28–31
7.8	28–31
7.9	29–32
8.0	29–33
8.1	29–33
8.2	30–34
8.3	30–34
8.4	31–35
8.5	31–35
8.6	31–35
8.7	31–35
8.8	31–36
8.9	32–36
9.0	33–37
9.1	33–37
9.2	35–38
9.3	35–38
9.4	35–39
9.5	35–39

* Only applicable to approximately ⅔ of normal pregnancies.[8,9]

younger fetus with the large BPD and incorrectly underestimated in the older fetus with a small BPD; the extent to which gestational age is incorrectly assigned varies from 7 to 11 days depending on whether the BPD is at the 75th or 95th percentile (Table 3–5).

If cephalometry is repeated during the interval of 31 to 33 weeks of pregnancy, the classification of fetal BPDs into large, average, and small growth patterns becomes possible (Table 3–6). The latter gestational interval is selected because it shows the maximal variation in large versus small fetal BPDs (Fig. 3–3). Additionally, in the presence of intrauterine growth retardation (IUGR), the majority of fetuses do not exhibit a reduction in cephalic size early in the third trimester of pregnancy, and their correct cephalic growth pattern can still be defined.[12]

The GASA chart (Table 3–6) shows the range in the BPD for fetuses with different growth patterns. Thus, by determining whether the second fetal BPD is large, average, or small, gestational age can be adjusted in relation to cephalic growth—thus the term growth-adjusted sonar age (GASA). For example, consider the same fetus with a BPD of 5.7 cm to whom a temporary mean gestational age of 23 weeks is

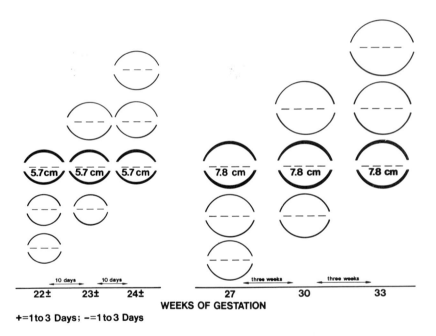

Figure 3–1. *Fetuses of the same gestational age have different BPD values. The difference is what accounts for the range in error of defining gestational age by BPD. By assigning all fetuses (regardless of cephalic size) a mean gestational age, the length of pregnancy is always incorrectly advanced in the younger fetus with a large head and underestimated in the older fetus with a small head; the range (± 2SD) in error is ± 10 to 11 days if BPD is obtained prior to 27 weeks' gestation but is ± 3 weeks if BPD is obtained in the third trimester of pregnancy. (From Sabbagha, R. E. and Hughey, M.: Standardization of sonar cephalometry and gestational age. Obstet. Gynecol., 52:405, 1978.)*

assigned. If cephalometry is repeated nine weeks later (i.e., at 32 weeks for a fetus with average cephalic size), the BPD will fall into one of three possible categories (shown in the GASA chart) (Table 3–6). For example, a BPD measurement of 8.1 cm would imply an average growth pattern, in which case gestational age is truly 32 weeks. On the

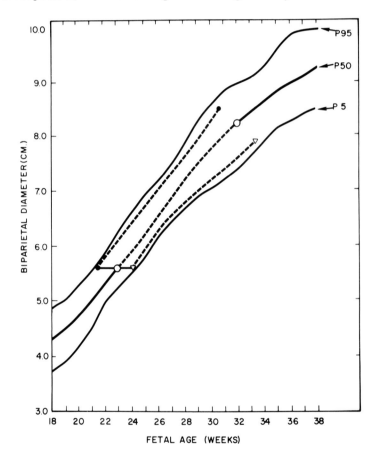

Figure 3–2.   *Percentile chart of sonar BPD at one-week intervals. Filled circle = young fetus (21+ weeks' gestation) with large BPD. Open circle = fetus with average BPD (23 weeks' gestation). Triangle = older fetus (24+ weeks' gestation) with small BPD. The growth pattern of the three fetuses is unknown from the first scan and a BPD of 5.7 is used to assign a mean gestational age (23 weeks) to all fetuses. Because each fetus maintains its respective growth pattern, a second BPD reading 9 weeks later defines the growth pattern for each fetus and leads to adjustment of gestational age accordingly (see text and Table 3–6). (From Sabbagha, R. E.: Intrauterine growth retardation: Antenatal diagnosis by ultrasound. Obstet. Gynecol., 52:252, 1978.)*

other hand, if the BPD is 8.6 cm, the fetus is placed in a large cephalic growth percentile. This means that its gestational age had been incorrectly advanced by at least 7 days and should be adjusted in accordance with its growth, i.e., reduced by one week. In other words, a growth-adjusted sonar age will now correctly define the length of pregnancy as 31 weeks. Likewise, if the BPD at 32 weeks is 7.8 cm, i.e., small, GASA will be 33 weeks.

In assigning fetuses a GASA, the following rules of thumb are helpful: (1) In the presence of a large BPD growth pattern, a GASA

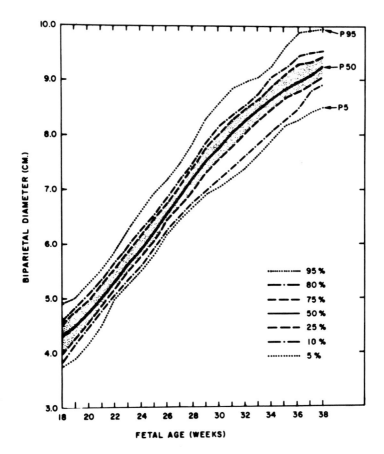

Figure 3–3. *Percentile chart of sonar BPD at one-week intervals. (From Sabbagha, R. E., Barton, F. B., Barton, B. A.: Sonar biparietal diameter I. Analysis of percentile growth differences in two normal populations using same methodology. Am. J. Obstet. Gynecol., 126:479, 1976.)*

Table 3–8. *Examples of Assignment of GASA*

| First Sonar 18 to 26 Weeks* | | | Second Sonar 30 to 33 Weeks† | | | | | | |
Date§	BPD (cm)	Average Fetal Age Accepted Temporarily (week)	Date§	Interval Between Scans (weeks)	Age of Average Fetus (weeks)	BPD Expected for Fetus of Average Size	BPD Obtained	GASA‡	BPD Percentile for GASA
8–12	4.2	18+	11–11	13	31+	8.0–8.2	8.2 (Same as expected)	31+ No change	25th–75th
1–10	5.8	23+	3–10	8+	32–	8.1–8.2	8.5 (Larger than expected)	31–, 1 week younger	75th–95th
2–15	5.1	21+	5–10	12	33+	8.5–8.6	9.1 (Much larger than expected)	32, Approximately 10 days younger	>95th
4–10	6.0	24	5–30	7+	31+	8.0–8.2	7.5 (Much smaller than expected)	33, Fetus is very small	<5th

BPD = biparietal diameter measured from outer to inner aspects of fetal head; + = plus 1–3 days; – = minus 1–3 days.

* First sonar is done prior to 26 weeks because of small variation in fetal age of ± 11 days.

† Second sonar: (1) Must be done between 30 to 33 weeks because of maximal variation in fetal BPD size in this interval and prior to onset of IUGR in most cases, and (2) must be done at least 6 weeks after first BPD.

‡ In comparison to fetuses with average BPDs those with larger BPDs are 1 week younger while those with smaller BPDs are 1 week older. If the BPD is very large or very small, the fetus is up to 11 days younger or older than an average fetus.

§ Gestation disc calculator is first rotated to show the date in relation to the 50th percentile fetal age accepted temporarily. If this fetal age is qualified by a plus or minus sign, the disc is rotated an average of 2 days to the left or right, respectively. The calculator will then show the date on which fetal age is approximately 30 to 33 weeks.

From Sabbagha, R.E., Hughey, M., and Depp, R.: Growth adjusted sonographic age: A simplified method. Obstet. Gynecol., *51*:384, 1978.

always reduces gestational age by at least one week; (2) in the presence of a small growth pattern, a GASA always advances gestational age by at least one week; and (3) in the presence of an average growth pattern, a GASA is the same as the mean gestational age. Four other illustrations of assigning fetuses a GASA are shown in Table 3–8.

GASA Chart. The GASA chart (Table 3–6) is statistically comparable to the composite mean BPD values derived from a number of reliable studies (see Chap. 2); however, it is preferable to use the GASA chart when serial cephalometry is performed at the appropriate intervals in gestation (17–24 and 31–33 weeks) for a variety of reasons: (1) precision with which the GASA chart is derived from menstrual data, shown in Figure 3–4; (2) the clear separation of fetuses into those with large, average, and small BPDs; (3) the placement of each fetus into a specific BPD percentile bracket by 32 weeks' gestation. In this way, assessment of continued BPD growth is possible in relation to each fetus's own potential rather than to a mean value derived from a general population of fetuses.[9]

Assignment of Gestational Age. Gestational age may be assigned by sonar in a number of ways, some more accurate and useful than others:

1. *CRL measurement of fetus* (accuracy of one measurement is ±4.7 days; ±2SD). This method is applicable until 12 to 13 weeks' gestation. A BPD reading should still be obtained by 31 to 33 weeks to assign each fetus a percentile growth bracket.

2. *Single BPD measurement obtained prior to 27 weeks' gestation* (accuracy ±11 days; ±2SD). The composite mean BPD table or the first part of the GASA chart may be used.

3. *Single BPD measurement obtained after 28 weeks' gestation* (accuracy ±3 weeks—90% of population). The gestational age of the fetus with average cephalic size may be reported in accordance with probability estimates (Table 3–7). In general, these reports are not applicable to ⅓ of fetuses—those with either large or small BPDs. The obstetrician dealing with high-risk gravidas should be careful in interpreting single BPD measurements obtained after 26 weeks' gestation because the incidence of fetuses with large cephalic size (as in maternal diabetes) or small cephalic size (as in growth retardation) is increased.

4. *Serial BPD measurements obtained at the appropriate intervals in gestation* (17–24 and 31–33 weeks) and used to define gestational age by the principle of GASA (accuracy ±1–3 days; ±2SD).

It should be emphasized that the onset of labor occurs within ±2 weeks of the expected date of delivery (EDD) in approximately 84% of

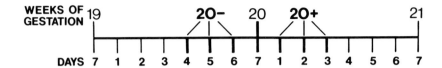

Figure 3–4. *In constructing the GASA chart showing the correlation between fetal BPDs and fetal age, the duration of pregnancy was ascertained from the first day of the last menstrual period as follows: (1) pregnancies which fell at the end of a whole week were assigned the exact fetal age corresponding to that week, e.g., 20 weeks; (2) pregnancies which fell 1 to 3 days beyond a completed week were labeled with a plus sign, e.g., 20+ weeks; and (3) pregnancies which fell 1 to 3 days short of a completed week were labeled with a minus sign, e.g., 20– weeks. (From Sabbagha, R. E. and Hughey, M.: Standardization of sonar cephalometry and gestational age. Obstet. Gynecol., 52:405, 1978.)*

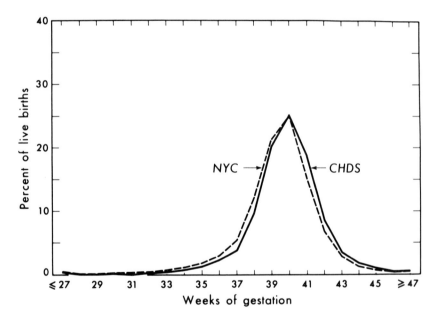

Figure 3–5. *Normal distribution of live births in relation to onset of labor in 420,000 pregnancies. Approximately 84% of gravidas deliver within ± 2 weeks of the menstrual expected date of delivery. (From Yerushalmy, J.: Relation of birth weight, gestational age and the rate of intrauterine growth to perinatal mortality. Clin. Obstet. Gynecol., 13:107, 1970.)*

women with known LMPs (Fig. 3–5). Thus, ''term'' extends from 38 to 42 weeks' gestation.

If gestational age is accurately defined by CRL or serial BPD (GASA) measurements, the onset of labor is still within ±2 weeks of the EDD in women who do not deliver prematurely or go past term. Many patients and even some physicians incorrectly assume that if gestational age is defined by either CRL values or GASA, delivery occurs within ±3 to 4 days of the EDD. This is not true because the range of ±3 to 4 days represents the 95% confidence limits of sonar assessment of gestational age and not the onset of labor.

References

1. Dewhurst, C. J., Beazley, J. M., and Campbell, S.: Assessment of the fetal maturity and dysmaturity. Am. J. Obstet. Gynecol., *113*:141, 1972.
2. Cowchock, F. S.: Use of alpha-feto protein in prenatal diagnosis. Clin. Obstet. Gynecol., *19*:871, 1976.
3. Merkatz, I., and Solomon, S.: The fetoplacental unit. Clin. Obstet. Gynecol., *13*:665, 1970.
4. Campbell, S.: The assessment of fetal development by diagnostic ultrasound. Clin. Perinatol., *1*:507, 1974.
5. Sabbagha, R.E.: Ultrasound in managing the high-risk pregnancy. *In* Management of the High-Risk Pregnancy. Edited by W. N. Spellacy. Baltimore, University Park Press, 1976.
6. Robinson, H. P., and Fleming, J. E. E.: A critical evaluation of sonar crown-rump length measurements. Br. J. Obstet. Gynaecol., *82*:702, 1975.
7. Drumm, J. E., Clinch, J., and MacKenzie, G.: The ultrasonic measurement of fetal crown-rump length as a method of assessing gestational age. Br. J. Obstet. Gynecol., *83*:417, 1976.
8. Sabbagha, R. E. et al.: Sonar BPD and fetal age: Definition of the relationship. Obstet. Gynecol., *43*:7, 1974.
9. Sabbagha, R. E. et al.: Sonar biparietal diameter: II. Predictive of three fetal growth patterns leading to a closer assessment of gestational age and neonatal weight. Am. J. Obstet. Gynecol., *126*:485, 1976.
10. Sabbagha, R. E., Turner, H. J., and Chez, R. A.: Sonar BPD growth standards in the rhesus monkey. Am. J. Obstet. Gynecol., *121*:371, 1975.
11. Sabbagha, R. E., Hughey, M., and Depp, R.: Growth adjusted sonographic age: A simplified method. Obstet. Gynecol., *51*:383, 1978.
12. Gruenwald, P.: Chronic fetal distress and placental insufficiency. Biol. Neonate, *5*:215, 1963.
13. Yerushalmy, J.: Relation of birth weight, gestational age and the rate of intrauterine growth to perinatal mortality. Clin. Obstet. Gynecol., *13*:107, 1970.

4

FETAL GROWTH

The distinction between normal and abnormal fetal growth by assessing maternal weight gain and growth of the uterine fundus is difficult.[1-4] A number of studies indicate that the clinical diagnosis of intrauterine growth retardation (IUGR), antenatally, is possible in approximately one-third of such pregnancies.[5,6] Sometimes IUGR is suspected when complications such as pre-eclampsia occur. However, more often than not, the diagnosis escapes the most astute obstetrician.

It is important to make the diagnosis of IUGR during the pregnancy or at least to identify gravidas who are at definite high risk of harboring an undergrown fetus, because a plan of management can then be outlined and followed. In this way, intelligent decisions based on a

Table 4-1. *Diagnosis of Intrauterine Growth Retardation by Serial Cephalometry—Five Studies*

	No. of IUGR Infants*	Correct IUGR Diagnosis by BPD (%)	Percent False-Positive	Percent False-Negative
Dewhurst et al.[8]	146	71	28	17
Whetham et al.[9]	23	70	—	30
Queenan et al.[10]	16	50	50	9
Arias[11]	12	43	57	—
Crane et al.[12]	9	100	36	—

* Below the 10th percentile of birth weight.[13]

Modified from Sabbagha, R.E.: Intrauterine growth retardation: Antenatal diagnosis by ultrasound. Obstet. Gynecol., *52*:252, 1978.

number of antenatal tests can be made regarding the most optimal time for delivery prior to the development of severe asphyxia—possibly leading to irreversible pathologic changes in the central nervous system or even to intrauterine fetal death.

In the last decade, many investigators evaluated the role of diagnostic ultrasound in the antenatal diagnosis of IUGR. Fetal cephalic, thoracic, and abdominal measurements have all been correlated (either singly or in combination) with fetal size. Recently, Gohari et al. related IUGR to a small total intrauterine volume (TIUV).[7]

Although the results of many studies have shown that sonography is superior to any other clinical or laboratory method for detecting IUGR, the degree of accuracy with which this is done, including false-positive and false-negative results, is variable (Table 4–1). This variability in results is related to a number of factors:

1. *Nonuniformity in ultrasound methodology* used to measure the biparietal diameter (BPD). As a result, the accuracy of some BPD readings may be questionable (see Chap. 1).

2. *Inaccurate dating* of some pregnancies, rendering interpretation of BPD growth data difficult.

3. *Evaluation* of BPD growth rate over a short period in pregnancy, such as 2, 4, or 6 weeks. During the third trimester of pregnancy, the difference in growth rate between fetuses with BPDs consistently falling at the 5th, 50th, and 95th percentiles is not statistically significant (Table 4–2). Additionally, by relating cephalic growth to a normal mean growth rate (expected from a general population of fetuses) the detection of IUGR is possible in a small proportion of fetuses (estimated at 5%).[14] The author believes that in a given pregnancy, definition of fetal growth pattern (large, average, or small) is much more useful for prediction of IUGR.[14]

It is interesting to note that the maxium difference in growth rate (0.6 cm) between fetuses with small and large BPDs is seen in the interval of 22 to 32 weeks' gestation—the interval used for assigning fetuses a growth-adjusted sonar age (Table 4–2).

4. *A less than optimal biologic correlation* between fetal cephalic, thoracic, or abdominal dimensions on the one hand and fetal weight on the other (Table 4–3).

Although the abdominal circumference (AC) is more closely predictive of fetal weight than any other parameter, the relationship (±450 g if the fetus is of average size) is still not sensitive enough for the absolute diagnosis of IUGR. For example, a term fetus estimated from the AC to weigh 3000 g may in fact turn out to be undergrown and

Table 4–2.   *BPD Growth Rate in Large, Average, and Small Fetuses over Short Intervals in the Third Trimester of Pregnancy*

	Size of Fetal BPD (Percentile)		
	Small 5	Average 50	Large 95
Week of Pregnancy:	28–32	28–32	28–32
BPD cm:	6.6–7.5	7.2–8.3	7.9–9.0
Growth rate cm:	0.9	1.1	1.1
Week of Pregnancy:	32–36	32–36	32–36
BPD cm:	7.5–8.3	8.3–9.0	9.0–9.7
Growth rate cm:	0.8	0.7	0.7
Week of Pregnancy:	30–36	30–36	30–36
BPD cm:	7.1–8.3	7.8–9.0	8.6–9.7
Growth rate cm:	1.2	1.2	1.1
Week of Pregnancy:	30–40	30–40	30–40
BPD cm:	7.1–8.9	7.8–9.5	8.6–10.1
Growth rate cm:	1.8	1.7	1.5
*Week of Pregnancy:	22–32	22–32	22–32
BPD cm:	4.9–7.5	5.3–8.3	5.8–9.0
Growth rate cm:	2.6	3	3.2

*Interval used for GASA.
BPD figures from Table 3–4 (Chap. 3).

weigh 2550 g. The predicted mean birth weight in relation to the AC is shown in Table 4–4.

The fact that the accuracy of birth weight from the AC is inversely related to actual weight, i.e., the smaller the fetal size, the greater the accuracy (Table 4–3), is important. Thus, in using the AC as a parameter for assessing fetal weight, a clear distinction between the small normal premature and the IUGR fetus should be made and can only be deduced if gestational age is accurately defined. For example, if the mean fetal weight predicted from the AC is 2000 g, the fetus will certainly be normal if the length of pregnancy is 33 weeks but undergrown if gestational age is 36 to 37 weeks.

5. *Correlating the tenth percentile of BPD with the tenth percentile of fetal body weight.* Statistically, undergrown fetuses are defined as those whose birth weights fall at or below the tenth percentile for a

Table 4–3. *Relationship of Biparietal Diameter (BPD) and Abdominal Circumference (AC) Measurements to Body Weights*

Study(s)	Parameters	Imaging Modality	Approximate Range in Weight (g±2SD)
2[20,21]	BPD	A	900
3[22–24]	BPD	B	650–750
1[6]	BPD	B–A	840
2[25,26]	BPD + Thorax	B	500
1[27]	Skull + Thoracic Area	B	±430
1[28]	BPD + AC	B	Related to actual weight: 212 at 1000 g 414 at 2000 g 636 at 3000 g 848 at 4000 g
1[29]	AC	B	Related to actual weight: 160 at 1000 g 290 at 2000 g 450 at 3000 g 590 at 4000 g

specific gestational week. Since neither the BPD nor the AC is a very sensitive index of birth weight, it is a fallacy to assume that when BPD or AC values fall at the tenth percentile, IUGR can be diagnosed with certainty. In fact, the author finds that all fetuses with BPDs below the 25th percentile (regardless of whether they are in the 20th or 5th percentile) are at the same high risk for IUGR, namely, 50%;[14] however, the other 50% are normal. The exact risk for IUGR in fetuses with AC values falling below the 25th percentile is still under study.

Fetal Growth Patterns and IUGR

The difficulties encountered in the assessment of fetal weight and IUGR by the conventional methods discussed may be circumvented if individual fetal growth patterns in all high-risk pregnancies are evaluated. In this way, a small group of fetuses who are at definite risk for

Table 4–4.   *Relationship Between Fetal Abdominal Circumference Measurements from 21 to 40 cm and Birth Weight Centiles*

Abdominal Circumference (cm)	Estimated Birth Weight Centiles (g)		
	5	50	95
21	780	900	1040
22	900	1030	1190
23	1030	1180	1360
24	1170	1340	1540
25	1320	1510	1730
26	1470	1690	1940
27	1640	1880	2150
28	1810	2090	2380
29	1990	2280	2610
30	2170	2490	2850
31	2350	2690	3080
32	2530	2900	3320
33	2710	3100	3550
34	2880	3290	3760
35	3030	3470	3970
36	3180	3640	4160
37	3310	3790	4330
38	3420	3920	4490
39	3510	4020	4610
40	3570	4100	4720

Modified from Campbell, S., and Wilkin, D.: Ultrasonic measurement of fetal abdominal circumference in estimation of fetal weight. Br. J. Obstet. Gynaecol., *82*:689, 1975.

IUGR can be identified and closely monitored by all available biophysical, bioelectric, and biochemical means to determine the most optimal time for delivery.

My colleagues and I recently showed that in the second half of pregnancy, in both monkey and human fetuses, cephalic growth for each fetus tends to fall consistently within one of three relatively narrow percentile ranks (Fig. 4–1) (see Chap. 3).

One advantage of this biologic behavior is the accurate definition of gestational age, early in the third trimester of pregnancy, by the principle of GASA (see Chap. 3). The other advantage is related to the fact that once BPDs are placed within a specific cephalic percentile rank by approximately 31 weeks' gestation, subsequent growth can be evaluated in relation to the potential expected for each fetus rather than to a mean value derived from a heterogeneous population of fetuses.

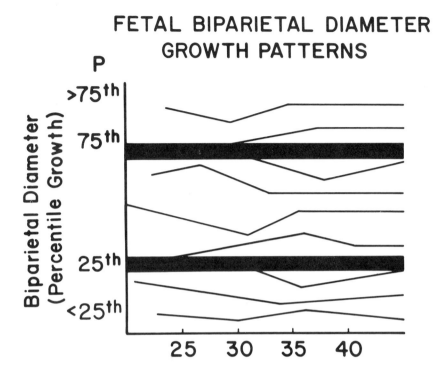

Figure 4–1. *Fetal biparietal diameter values normally remain in the same percentile bracket: large (>75th P), average (25th–75th P), and small (<25th P). (From Sabbagha, R. E. et al.: Sonar biparietal diameter II. Predictive of three fetal growth patterns leading to a closer assessment of gestational age and neonatal weight. Am. J. Obstet. Gynecol., 126:485, 1976.)*

The author has defined the precise risk for IUGR in fetuses who conform to two basic cephalic growth groups. The first group consists of those who maintain the BPD in either a large, average, or small pattern (the majority) and the second, those in whom the BPD drops from an upper to a lower percentile bracket (e.g., large to average or average to small).

IUGR IN FETUSES WHO MAINTAIN BPD GROWTH

Asymmetric IUGR. The risk for IUGR in fetuses who consistently maintain a large or average BPD growth profile is 3.5% and 10%, respectively (Fig. 4–2). Obviously, the affected fetus in any of these

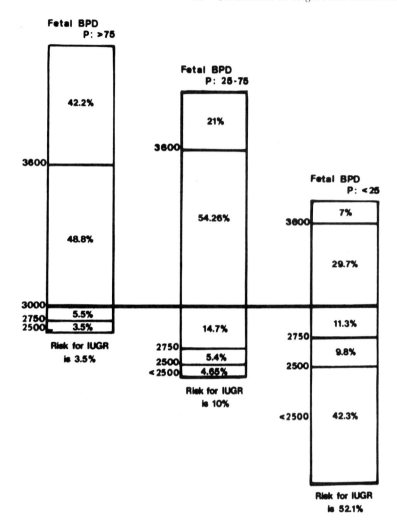

Figure 4–2. *Data derived from 463 high-risk gravidas defining the risk for IUGR in relation to BPD growth profile. (From Sabbagha, R. E.: Intrauterine growth retardation: Antenatal diagnosis by ultrasound. Obstet. Gynecol., 52:252, 1978.)*

two groups is asymmetrically undergrown because cephalic size falls within an upper percentile rank while body weight is ≤ the tenth percentile.

There are two interesting facets to this type of asymmetric IUGR. First, the prognosis, based at least on the number of brain cells (to the exclusion of the possible hazards of asphyxia), is expected to be better than that in symmetric IUGR.[15-18] In symmetric IUGR, the insult is prolonged, resulting in a proportional reduction of both cephalic and body size. Second, fetuses in the asymmetric group cannot be differentiated by serial cephalometry alone because cephalic size falls within the normal range (Fig. 4–3). However, an ultrasonically derived AC measurement by 36 weeks' gestation is likely to delineate the asymmetrically undergrown fetus (exact probability under study) because the BPD and AC fall in different percentile (P) ranks: BPD is > 25th P and AC is < 25th P. Placing the BPD and AC in specific percentile categories may obviate the need to measure the circumference of the

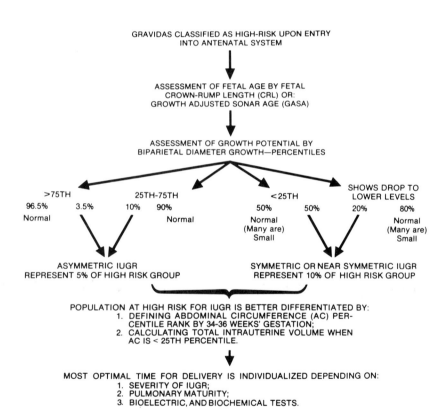

Figure 4–3. *Steps in evaluating high-risk pregnancies upon entry into an antenatal system of care. Note: Approximately 15% of this high-risk pregnant population delivered IUGR fetuses; of these two-thirds were symmetrically or near symmetrically undergrown and one-third represented asymmetric growth retardation.*

Table 4–5.   *Head to Abdomen (H/A) Ratios (Mean and +2SD) in Relation To Gestational Age*[19]

Weeks' Gestation	H/A Ratios	
	Mean	+2SD
28	1.13	1.21
32	1.08	1.17
34	1.04	1.13
36	1.02	1.12
38	0.99	1.06
40	0.97	1.05

fetal head to determine the head-to-abdomen (H/A) ratio suggested by Campbell and Thoms.[19] These investigators showed that by 36 weeks' gestation, approximately 70% of asymmetric IUGR fetuses maintain a H/A ratio ≥2SD above the mean value (Table 4–5). In contrast, the H/A ratio is ≤1 between 36 and 38 weeks of gestation in normal fetuses.

Symmetric IUGR. The risk for IUGR in the fetus who consistently maintains a BPD growth profile below the 25th percentile is approximately 50% (Fig. 4–2).[14] The affected fetus in this group exhibits symmetric or near symmetric growth retardation because cephalic size is below the 25th percentile and body weight is ≤ the 10th percentile. Approximately two-thirds of IUGR fetuses are symmetrically or near symmetrically undergrown (Figs. 4–2 and 4–3).[14]

Although as a group fetuses with BPDs falling below the 25th percentile are identified by serial cephalometry and are at high risk (50%) for IUGR (Fig. 4–3), preliminary data indicate that the affected fetus may be singled out if the ultrasonic measurement of the abdominal circumference also falls below the 25th percentile (exact probability under study, see below).

IUGR IN FETUSES WHO SHOW A DROP IN BPD GROWTH

The risk for IUGR in fetuses who cannot maintain an average growth pattern and who drop to lower percentile brackets is 20%.[14] This group constitutes a small proportion of high-risk pregnancies (approximately 5%),[14] and the affected fetuses can be either symmetrically or asymmetrically undergrown.

GROWTH PATTERNS BY BPD AND AC

If the cephalic percentile rank (derived from serial BPDs; Chap. 3, Table 3–7) is used in conjunction with the abdominal circumference percentile rank (derived from one or two AC values at 34–36 weeks' gestation, Table 4–6), fetal growth falls into one of nine possible patterns (Table 4–7). In this way, the risk of a fetus being large for gestational age (LGA) or small for gestational age (SGA) can be better delineated. For example, fetuses at definite risk of being LGA are likely to fall in pattern no. 1 (Table 4–7); fetuses at definite risk for asymmetric IUGR are those in patterns 3 and 6 (Table 4–7); fetuses at definite risk for symmetric IUGR are those in pattern 9 (Table 4–7).

Table 4–6. *Fetal Abdominal Circumference Measurements (cm)**

Weeks of Gestation	PERCENTILE								
	2.5	5	10	25	50	75	80	95	97.5
18	9.8	10.3	10.9	11.9	13.1	14.2	14.5	15.9	16.4
19	11.1	11.6	12.3	13.3	14.4	15.6	15.9	17.2	17.8
20	12.1	12.6	13.3	14.3	15.4	16.6	16.9	18.2	18.8
21	13.7	14.2	14.8	15.9	17.0	18.1	18.4	19.8	20.3
22	14.7	15.2	15.8	16.9	18.0	19.1	19.4	20.8	21.3
23	16.0	16.5	17.1	18.2	19.3	20.4	20.7	22.1	22.6
24	17.2	17.7	18.3	19.4	20.5	21.6	21.9	23.3	23.8
25	18.0	18.5	19.1	20.2	21.3	22.4	22.7	24.1	24.6
26	18.8	19.3	19.9	21.0	22.1	23.2	23.5	24.9	25.4
27	20.4	20.9	21.5	22.6	23.7	24.8	25.1	26.5	27.0
28	22.0	22.5	23.1	24.2	25.3	26.4	26.7	28.1	28.6
29	23.6	24.1	24.7	25.8	26.9	28.0	28.3	29.7	30.2
30	24.1	24.6	25.2	26.3	27.4	28.5	28.8	30.2	30.7
31	24.7	25.2	25.8	26.9	28.0	29.1	29.4	30.8	31.3
32	25.4	25.9	26.5	27.6	28.7	29.8	30.1	31.5	32.0
33	25.7	26.2	26.8	27.9	29.0	30.1	30.4	31.8	32.3
34	26.8	27.3	27.9	29.0	30.1	31.2	31.5	32.9	33.4
35	28.9	29.4	30.0	31.1	32.2	33.3	33.6	35.0	35.5
36	30.0	30.5	31.1	32.2	33.3	34.4	34.7	36.1	36.6
37	31.1	31.6	32.2	33.3	34.4	35.5	35.8	37.2	37.7
38	32.4	32.9	33.5	34.6	35.7	36.8	37.1	38.5	39.0
39	32.6	33.1	33.7	34.8	35.9	37.0	37.3	38.7	39.2
40	32.8	33.3	33.9	35.0	36.1	37.2	37.5	38.9	39.4
41	33.8	34.3	34.9	36.0	37.1	38.2	38.5	39.9	40.4

* Circumference measurements are obtained from the outer aspect of the fetal abdomen at the area of the liver that shows the ductus venosus.[30]

Table 4–7.   *Fetal Growth Patterns by Serial Biparietal Diameter (BPD) and Abdominal Circumference (AC) Measurements*

Fetal Growth Pattern	Serial BPD Growth Pattern (Percentile)	AC at 36 weeks' Gestation (Percentile)
1	>75th	>75th
2	>75th	25th–75th
3	>75th	<25th
4	25th–75th	>75th
5	25th–75th	25th–75th
6	25th–75th	<25th
7	<25th	>75th
8	<25th	25th–75th
9	<25th	<25th

LGA fetus is likely to fall in growth pattern no. 1.
Asymmetric IUGR fetus is likely to fall in growth patterns 3 and 6.
Symmetric IUGR fetus is likely to fall in growth pattern no. 9.

Table 4–8.   *Total Intrauterine Volume (TIUV) at 1.5 SD* Below Mean in Relation to Gestational Age*[7]

Weeks' Gestation	TIUV, 1.5 SD Below Mean
16	450
18	600
20	750
22	900
24	1100
26	1250
28	1500
30	1750
32	2000
34	2350
36	2550
38	2850
40	3000

* Figures rounded to approximate numbers. TIUV in 75% of growth-retarded fetuses falls below 1.5 SD of mean value in relation to a specific week of gestation.

TIUV is derived by multiplication of: sonar-derived uterine length × width × depth × 0.5233.[7]

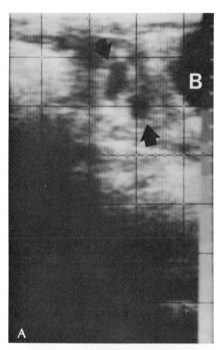

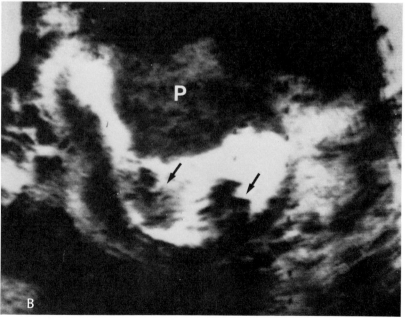

Figure 4–4. *A, Twin gestational sacs (arrows) with no fetuses (blighted ova) obtained by using real-time apparatus. B = bladder. B, Transverse scan of twin fetuses (arrows) approximately 9 to 10 weeks' gestation. P = placenta.*

Measurement of total intrauterine volume (TIUV) (Table 4–8) may also be helpful in confirming IUGR in growth patterns 3, 6, and 9.

Fetal Growth Evaluation

In evaluating fetal growth it is important first to define gestational age (by fetal CRL or by BPDs utilizing the principle of GASA). Second, the fetus should be placed in an upper, average, or small cephalic percentile bracket by 32 weeks' gestation. Finally BPD and AC percentile ranks, if assigned between the 35th and 37th weeks of pregnancy, provide information regarding the specific growth pattern for each fetus. In particular, the risk for symmetric or asymmetric IUGR may be defined (Fig. 4–3). Pregnancies at high risk for altered fetal growth should then be evaluated by a variety of antenatal tests for determination of the most optimal time for delivery.

Assessment of gestational age (by CRL or GASA methods) and of individual fetal growth is also essential for twins (Fig. 4–4). In this way disparate growth may be identified early and the benefit of treatment (e.g., bed rest) may be evaluated by serial sonar measurements of cephalic and abdominal dimensions.[31,32] In general, the mean BPD of twin fetuses is below that of singletons near term, and divergent growth of approximately 6 mm may indicate severe compromise in one twin.[32] No data, however, are available to show the frequency of fetuses with large, average, or small cephalic dimensions.

The question pertaining to the most optimal time for delivery of an SGA fetus is not yet scientifically answered. The management of each fetus should be individualized, depending on the duration of growth retardation, severity of maternal medical complications, and the results of the biophysical and biochemical tests.

Some obstetricians feel that when the diagnosis of IUGR is made, there is no need to delay delivery appreciably beyond 36 weeks' gestation if pulmonary maturity is attained then.[33] Others believe that delivery should not be effected unless bioelectric and biochemical tests are abnormal.[34]

References

1. Lind, T.: The estimation of fetal growth and development. Br. J. Hosp. Med., *3*:501, 1970.

2. Johnson, R. W., and Toshach, C. E.: Estimation of fetal weight using longitudinal mensuration. Am. J. Obstet. Gynecol., 68:891, 1954.
3. Beazley, J. M., and Underhill, R. A.: Fallacy of the fundal height. Br. Med. J., 4:404, 1970.
4. Ong, H. C., and Sen, D. K.: Clinical estimation of fetal weight. Am. J. Obstet. Gynecol., 112:877, 1972.
5. Mann, L. I., Tejani, N. A., and Weiss, R. R.: Antenatal diagnosis and management of the small-for-gestational age fetus. Am. J. Obstet. Gynecol., 120:995, 1974.
6. Campbell, S.: The assessment of fetal development by diagnostic ultrasound. Clin. Perinatol., 1:507, 1974.
7. Gohari, P., Berkowitz, R. L., and Hobbins, J. C.: Prediction of intrauterine growth retardation by determination of total intrauterine volume. Am. J. Obstet. Gynecol., 127:255, 1977.
8. Dewhurst, C. J., Beazley, J. M., and Campbell, S.: Assessment of fetal maturity and dysmaturity. Am. J. Obstet. Gynecol., 113:141, 1972.
9. Whetham, J. C. G., Muggah, H., and Davidson, S.: Assessment of intrauterine growth retardation by diagnostic ultrasound. Am. J. Obstet. Gynecol., 125:577, 1976.
10. Queenan, J. T. et al.: Diagnostic ultrasound for detection of intrauterine growth retardation. Am. J. Obstet. Gynecol., 124:865, 1976.
11. Arias, F.: The diagnosis and management of intrauterine growth retardation. Obstet. Gynecol., 49:293, 1977.
12. Crane, J. P., Kopta, M. M., Welt, S. I., and Sauvage, J. P.: Abnormal fetal growth patterns: Ultrasonic diagnosis and management. Obstet. Gynecol., 50:205, 1977.
13. Battaglia, F. C., and Lubchenco, L. O.: A practical classification of newborn infants by weight and gestational age. J. Pediatr., 71:159, 1967.
14. Sabbagha, R. E.: Intrauterine growth retardation: Antenatal diagnosis by ultrasound. Obstet. Gynecol., 52:252, 1978.
15. Wigglesworth, J. S.: Experimental growth retardation in the foetal rat. J. Pathol. Bacteriol., 88:1, 1964.
16. Winick, M., Coscia, A., and Noble, A.: Cellular growth in human placenta: I. Normal placental growth. Pediatrics, 39:248, 1967.
17. Winick, M., and Noble, A.: Quantitative changes in DNA, RNA, and protein during prenatal and postnatal growth in the rat. Develop. Biol., 12:451, 1965.
18. Naeye, R. L.: Prenatal organ and cellular growth with various chromosomal disorders. Biol. Neonate, 11:248, 1967.
19. Campbell, S., and Thoms, A.: Ultrasonic measurement of fetal abdominal circumference ratio in the assessment of growth retardation. Br. J. Obstet. Gynaecol., 84:165, 1977.
20. Willocks, J., Donald, I., Duggan, T. C., and Day, N.: Foetal cephalometry by ultrasound. Br. J. Obstet. Gynaecol., 71:11, 1964.
21. Kohorn, E. T.: An evaluation of ultrasonic fetal cephalometry. Am. J. Obstet. Gynecol., 97:553, 1967.
22. Stocker, J., Mawad, R., Deleon, A., and Desjardins, P.: Ultrasonic cephalometry— Its use in estimating fetal weight. Obstet. Gynecol., 45:275, 1974.
23. Sabbagha, R.E., and Turner, H. J.: Methodology of B-scan sonar cephalometry with electronic calipers and correlation with fetal birth weight. Obstet. Gynecol., 40:74, 1972.
24. Ianniruberto, A., and Gibbons, J. M.: Predicting fetal weight by ultrasonic B-scan cephalometry: An improved technic with disappointing results. Obstet. Gynecol., 37:689, 1971.

25. Thompson, H. E., and Makowski, E. L.: Birth weight and gestational age. Obstet. Gynecol., *37*:44, 1971.
26. Hansman, M.: Ultraschallbiometrie in II und III Trimester der Schwangerschaft. Gynaekologe, *9*:133, 1976.
27. Lunt, R., and Chard, T.: A new method for estimation of fetal weight in late pregnancy by ultrasonic scanning. Br. J. Obstet. Gynaecol., *83*:1, 1976.
28. Warsof, S. L., Gohari, P., Berkowitz, R. L., and Hobbins, J. C.: The estimation of fetal weight by computer-assisted analysis. Am. J. Obstet. Gynecol., *128*:881, 1977.
29. Campbell, S., and Wilkin, D.: Ultrasonic measurement of fetal abdominal circumference in estimation of fetal weight. Br. J. Obstet. Gynaecol., *82*:689, 1975.
30. Tamura, R., and Sabbagha, R. E.: Percentile ranks of Sonar fetal abdominal circumference measurements. Work in progress.
31. Houlton, M. C. C.: Divergent biparietal growth rates in twin pregnancies. Obstet. Gynecol., *49*:542, 1977.
32. Haney, A. F., Crenshaw, C. M., and Dempsey, P. J.: Significance of biparietal diameter differences between twins. Obstet. Gynecol., *51*:609, 1968.
33. Tejani, N., Mann, L. I., and Weiss, R. R.: Antenatal diagnosis and management of the small-for-gestational-age fetus. Obstet. Gynecol., *47*:31, 1976.
34. Cetrulo, C., and Freeman, R.: Bioelectric evaluation in intrauterine growth retardation. Clin. Obstet. Gynecol., *20*:4, 979, 1977.

5

ABNORMALITIES OF PREGNANCY

Abnormalities of pregnancy may involve (1) amniotic fluid, (2) fetus, (3) placenta, and (4) pelvic masses. This chapter deals with the echo pattern in each of these groups, except placenta (see Chap. 6), and illustrates the usefulness of sonography to the clinician in the day-to-day management of pregnant women.

Amniotic Fluid

It is interesting to note that gravidas are usually referred for an ultrasound study not so much to rule out amniotic fluid abnormalities, but rather to investigate the reason why fundal height is larger or smaller than menstrual dates—physical findings that may be due to a number of diagnostic possibilities listed in Table 5–1.

Determination of the exact volume of amniotic fluid by sonography is time consuming and may be imprecise. However, the sonographer can readily appreciate two abnormal entities: polyhydramnios and oligohydramnios.

Polyhydramnios. In polyhydramnios, the echogram shows the uterus to be overdistended with amniotic fluid (a large echo-free area is seen) (Fig. 5–1). In addition, small circular structures (blotches) representing sections of fetal extremities are visualized at some distance from each other (Fig. 5–1); in the absence of these echoes, particularly in the last trimester of pregnancy, the diagnosis of achondroplasia should be considered and verified by plain film of the abdomen.[7] In polyhydram-

Table 5–1.   *Differential Diagnosis of Physical Findings When Fundal Height Is Larger or Smaller Than Menstrual Dates*

Fundal Height vs. Menstrual Dates	
Fundal height larger than menstrual dates	Fundal height smaller than menstrual dates
Inaccurate menstrual dates*	Inaccurate menstrual dates*
Polyhydramnios	Oligohydramnios
Fetal congenital anomalies	Fetal congenital anomalies
Fetus large for gestational age (LGA)	Fetus small for gestational age (SGA)
Multiple pregnancy	Usually single pregnancy
Molar pregnancy	Molar pregnancy unlikely
Pelvic mass (inaccessible to examination)	——

* Menstrual dates are inaccurate in up to 40% of gravidas.[13,14]

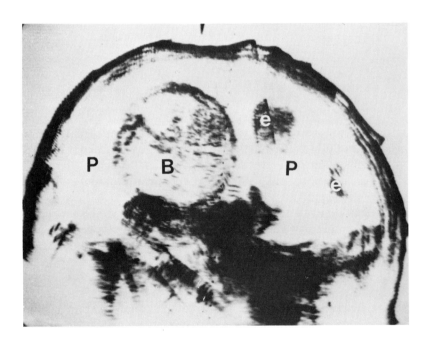

Figure 5–1.   *Transverse scan showing polyhydramnios (P). Note cross section of fetal body (B) and sections of fetal extremities (e) separated from each other.*

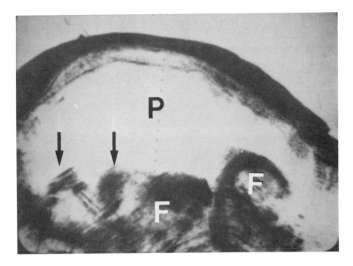

Figure 5–2.   *Longitudinal scan with marked polyhydramnios (P) at 28 weeks' gestation. Note fetus (F) lying along posterior aspect of uterine wall. Extremities (arrow) can be visualized and achondroplasia ruled out despite absence of sections of fetal extremities floating in fluid (Fig. 5–1).*

nios, the fetus is most often seen close to the posterior uterine wall rather than floating within the amniotic fluid (Fig. 5–2).

The finding of polyhydramnios is significant because it directs the sonographer to search for fetal congenital anomalies, and the obstetrician to rule out diabetes mellitus.

Oligohydramnios. "True" oligohydramnios (i.e., not secondary to premature rupture of membranes or postmaturity) is a rare entity. It may be associated with a variety of fetal congenital anomalies, most commonly renal agenesis. Moreover, adhesions between the amnion and parts of the fetus may cause serious musculoskeletal deformities.

In oligohydramnios, the fetus is usually seen in a "bent over" position, and because of the absence of fluid, transmission of sound is less than optimal, resulting in poor visualization of fetal internal structures. Nonetheless, major congenital anomalies may still be recognized sonographically.

Fetal Abnormality

Mass Screening. Antenatal sonar testing for detection of fetal abnormality is not presently performed on a routine basis in the United States or in most parts of the world. One of the potential benefits of a mass screening program is early (second trimester) diagnosis of some major congenital anomalies. As a result, the gravida and her partner would have the option of terminating the pregnancy prior to the attainment of fetal viability. However, mass screening by ultrasound is not feasible at this time. The reasons pertain to risk-benefit and cost-benefit ratios, as well as to the availability of sufficiently trained personnel.[1]

Risk- and Cost-Benefit Ratios. To date, exposure to pulsed ultrasound has not been shown to produce adverse fetal effects.[2-6] Yet, some researchers argue that long-term ill effects of sonic energy, even at the low levels used diagnostically ($10–20 \text{ mW/cm}^2$), have not been defined. Thus, sonography cannot be declared unequivocally safe and should only be used in the presence of medical or obstetric high-risk factors. The high-risk criteria that should lead the obstetrician to request an ultrasound examination to rule out some congenital anomalies are listed in Table 5–2.

In terms of the cost-benefit ratio, it also appears that the number of anomalies (or yield) detected in a mass screening venture would be small and that the yield does not justify the present-day cost of the examination.

Qualified Personnel. Despite recent advances in sonar technology, the diagnosis of fetal congenital anomalies requires extensive skill and experience on the part of the sonographer. In addition, both gray-scale

Table 5–2. *High-Risk Criteria Used as Indications for Ultrasound Study to Rule Out Congenital Anomalies*

Fundal height larger than menstrual date
Fundal height smaller than menstrual date
History of congenital anomalies
Maternal diabetes mellitus
Maternal age $\geqslant 35$ years
High serum AFP*
Bleeding in early pregnancy
Exposure to drugs or roentgen rays in early weeks of pregnancy

* AFP = α-fetoprotein

and real-time equipment should be at the disposal of the ultrasound specialist to enable him to make definitive diagnoses. Even then, some major anomalies such as meningomyelocele and duodenal atresia may still have to be confirmed by amniography.

FETAL ABNORMALITY IN EARLY PREGNANCY

During the last few years vast experience has been gained in evaluating early pregnancy by ultrasound. Initially, research was directed toward study of the shape, size, and uterine location of the early gestational sac.[7,8] It soon became apparent that this approach could not be reliably used to assess the status of pregnancy because the gestational sac varies in shape not only between longitudinal and transverse scans, but also in relation to the degree of bladder distention. The gestational sac is first visualized by 5 to 6 weeks after the first day of the last menstrual period.

Recently, emphasis has shifted toward the fetus. Development of gray-scale and real-time imaging has made it possible not only to visualize the longitudinal axis of the fetus (for measurement of crown-rump length) but also to observe the fetus directly, for evidence of body or heart motion, or both—as early as 7 to 8 weeks' gestation,[9] i.e., when the fetus is first visualized sonographically.

The sonographic differential diagnosis of early intrauterine pregnancy includes (1) normal pregnancy; (2) inaccurate dates; (3) blighted ovum; (4) missed abortion; and (5) hydatidiform mole.

Normal Pregnancy. If, in the presence of vaginal bleeding, a live fetus is seen by real-time sonar and the CRL correlates with menstrual age, the patient and the physician can be assured of the outcome of pregnancy because the prognosis is favorable in over 80% of such women.[10-12] This finding is indeed significant because it implies that fetal wastage occurs early, i.e., prior to the stage when fetal motion can first be detected by sonar (at 7–8 weeks' gestation).

Inaccurate Dates. If on the first scan the fetus is alive but smaller than dates, two possibilities exist. Menstrual dates may be inaccurate, or fetal growth may be abnormal—not likely at this early stage. Thus, the gravida is asked to return for serial sonar studies (weekly for 3 weeks) to define gestational age and evaluate fetal growth by fetal CRL measurements (see Chap. 3).

Blighted Ovum. Blighted ovum is the term applied to a fertilized ovum in which development is arrested early in pregnancy and only a

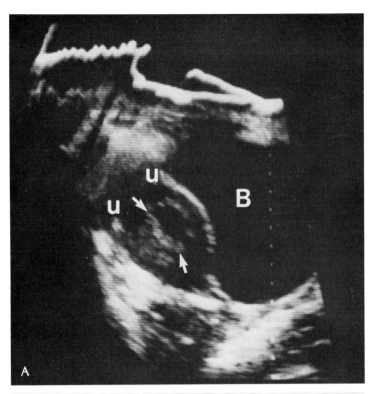

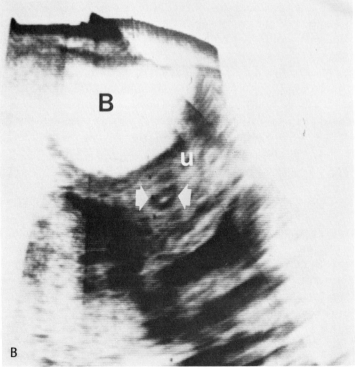

rudimentary fetus, if any, is identified. This entity is suspected when the fetus cannot be visualized and the gestational sac is either small or appropriate for dates (Figs. 5–3, 5–4). In the presence of a small "empty" sac, menstrual dates may be inaccurate and the pregnancy may be small but normal (Fig. 5–3). Serial studies are therefore requested to differentiate these two conditions. If, on the other hand, the sac is large and "empty," the diagnosis of blighted ovum is made. In blighted ovum, growth of the gestational sac may continue in some cases, albeit at a slow rate. Additionally, in many such gravidas the urinary chorionic gonadotropin (UCG) may remain positive until the end of the first trimester of pregnancy.

Missed Abortion. Missed abortion is the term used to denote early fetal demise, usually by 6 to 7 weeks' gestation. In these cases, a fetal pole is still recognized by sonar, but no fetal motion is visualized by real-time imaging. The differentiation between missed abortion and hydatidiform mole is discussed elsewhere (see Chap. 6).

It should be emphasized that the diagnosis of fetal demise, whether early or late in pregnancy, is best made by real-time imaging. In this way fetal body and heart motion, if present, is visually appreciated, and there is no room for error. The sign pertaining to collapse of the fetal head in intrauterine fetal death is not only late in appearance but may also be nonspecific.

FETAL ABNORMALITY IN MID AND LATE PREGNANCY

The fetal congenital anomalies that can be diagnosed by ultrasound in mid and late pregnancy (Table 5–3) are now discussed.

Neural Tube Defects. In the latter part of pregnancy, *hydrocephalus* may be readily recognized because the fetal head is large in relation to

Figure 5–3. *A, Longitudinal scan obtained by real-time imaging. The gestational sac (arrows) is approximately 6 weeks' size. No fetus is seen—a finding which may be normal if dates are accurate and consistent with size. However, this finding is abnormal if patient is 8 weeks by menstrual dates. A repeat scan is necessary (in 7–14 days) and if a live fetus is seen 80% of such pregnancies will be normal. B = bladder; u = uterus. B, Transverse gray-scale scan. A 5-week gestational sac is seen (arrows). Repeat examination in 2 weeks is necessary to differentiate blighted ovum or missed abortion from normal pregnancy. B = bladder; u = uterus.*

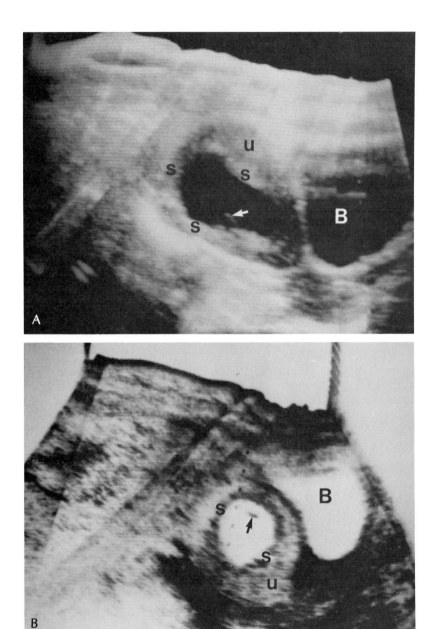

Figure 5–4. *A, Longitudinal gray-scale (white on black) plane showing large gestational sac (s) filling the uterus (u). However, a rudimentary fetus is seen (arrow) consistent with a diagnosis of blighted ovum. B = bladder. B, Longitudinal gray-scale (black on white) plane showing large 8- to 10-week gestation sac (s) filling the uterus (u). Note rudimentary fetus (arrow). Diagnosis: blighted ovum.*

Table 5-3. *Fetal Congenital Anomalies Detected by Diagnostic Ultrasound*

Neural tube defects	—Hydrocephaly
	—Anencephaly
	—Spina bifida
	—Meningomyelocele
Cardiac	—Bradycardia*
Gastrointestinal	—Bowel obstruction
	—Fetal ascites
Renal	—Multicystic kidneys
	—Renal agenesis
	—Bladder obstruction
Extremities	—Short extremities
	—Achondroplasia

* Related to possible abnormal neuromuscular developement of myocardium.

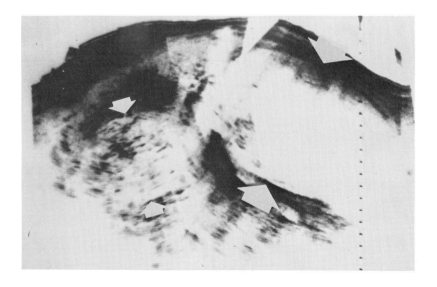

Figure 5-5. *Hydrocephalic fetus at term. Note body size (small arrows) vs. cephalic size (large arrows). Lateral walls of ventricular system are not seen because they are close to skull tables.*

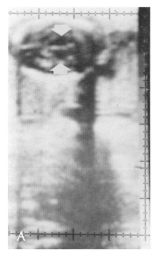

Figure 5–6. *A, Real-time image of fetal head (approximately 22 weeks' gestation). Note that lateral walls of ventricular system (arrows) do not normally extend more than halfway between midline echo and skull tables. B, Gray-scale image of fetal head (approximately 25 weeks' gestation) also showing normal ventricles (between arrows).*

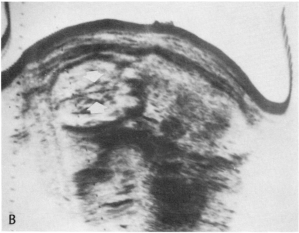

the fetal body. This increase in size is attributed to marked dilatation of the ventricular system of the brain; in this advanced state the lateral walls of the ventricles are not visualized because they are proximal to the skull table (Fig. 5–5).

Normally, the ventricles are sonographically visualized by both real-time and gray-scale imaging from 14 weeks' gestation (Figs. 5–5 and 5–6). Although ventricular size in fetuses of different gestational ages has not been firmly established, Campbell reports that the ventricles become smaller over a short period in the second trimester of pregnancy. Specifically, by 15 weeks' gestation, the walls of the ventricles normally extend to two-thirds of the distance between the midline cephalic echo and outer skull tables (as seen by sonar), whereas by 17 weeks, the walls recede to less than half that distance.[15]

Using these criteria, he correctly diagnosed hydrocephalus in four cases at 17 weeks' gestation. Interestingly, in all four fetuses, the BPD was still normal, indicating that ventricular dilatation actually precedes cephalic enlargement.

The diagnosis of hydrocephalus should not be made just because the BPD is large, for example, 10 or 11 cm. Rather, BPD and fetal trunk should be compared to the upper limits of normal for gestational age (see Chap. 4). If BPD is much larger than trunk size, the fetus may be hydrocephalic.

The sonar diagnosis of *anencephalus* can also be made as early as 14 to 15 weeks' gestation. In this abnormality, real-time scanning is particularly useful because it permits immediate recognition of the longitudinal lie of the fetus and enables the sonographer to compare cephalic with trunk dimensions (Fig. 5–7). The diagnosis of anencephaly may also be confirmed by a flat film of the abdomen.

The diagnosis of *spina bifida* is also possible. The spinal canal is best visualized by real-time sonar because the transducer is attached to a cord and may be manipulated to the appropriate angle for visualization

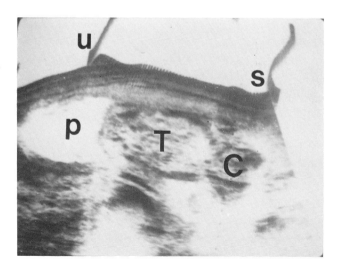

Figure 5–7. *Longitudinal scan of 20-week anencephalic fetus. Note small cephalic outline (C) vs. normal trunk. s = symphysis pubis; u = umbilicus; p = polyhydramnios; T = fetal trunk.*

Table 5–4.   *Relative Accuracy of Ultrasound (U/S) and α-Fetoprotein (AFP)* in the Early Diagnosis of 28 Neural Tube Defects*

	Correct Diagnosis		Missed Diagnosis		False Positive Diagnosis	
	U/S	AFP	U/S	AFP	U/S	AFP
Anencephaly	13	13	0	0	0	0
Spina Bifida	10	13	3	0	0	4
Encephalocele	2	2	0	0	0	0
Total	25	28	3	0	0	4

* AFP in amniotic fluid.

From Campbell, S.: Early prenatal diagnosis of neural tube defects by ultrasound. Clin. Obstet. Gynecol., *20*:357, 1976.

of the spine (see Chap. 1). Normally, the spinal canal appears as a hollow tube and may have to be displayed in two parts, particularly if photographs of real-time images are obtained (Fig. 5–8).

The spinal canal should be thoroughly scanned in both longitudinal and transverse planes. Campbell prefers to base his diagnosis on multiple transverse scans, especially for detecting a small spina bifida. He describes the defect as a U-shaped deformity.[15]

A comparison of the accuracy of ultrasound and α-fetoprotein (AFP) for antenatal detection of neural tube defects is shown in Table 5–4. It is apparent that the diagnosis of spina bifida situated at a level below the fourth lumbar vertebra can be missed in a small percentage of fetuses examined by ultrasound. However, AFP levels are falsely elevated in some patients and may lead the gravida to terminate the pregnancy unnecessarily.

In amniotic fluid, elevated levels of AFP are attributed to: (1) neural tube defect; (2) length of pregnancy less advanced than estimated by menstrual dates; (3) gastrointestinal anomalies; and (4) false positive levels (twins, missed abortion). To differentiate these possibilities, it appears that when a neural tube defect is suspected, gravidas should be examined by both ultrasound and AFP assays. Sonar may not only confirm or rule out a neural tube defect suspected from a high AFP determination, but also define gestational age and insure proper interpretation of AFP data.

Meningomyelocele can be diagnosed by both sonar and AFP levels. The author recently described a case of occipitothoracic meningocele diagnosed by sonar at 22 weeks' gestation.[16] The gravida and her partner elected to terminate the pregnancy (Fig. 5–9).

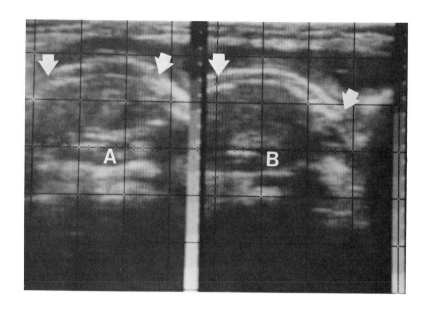

Figure 5–8. *Photograph of fetal spine (hollow tube—arrows) displayed by real-time. A = upper part of spine; B = lower part of spine.*

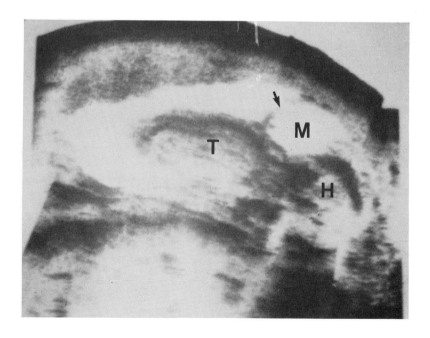

Figure 5–9. *Longitudinal scan of 22-week fetus with occipitothoracic meningocele (M). Note sac wall (arrow). H = fetal head; T = fetal trunk.*

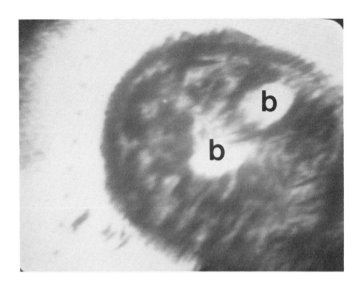

Figure 5–10. *Cross section of fetal abdominal circumference with double bubble sign (b & b) due to duodenal obstruction.*

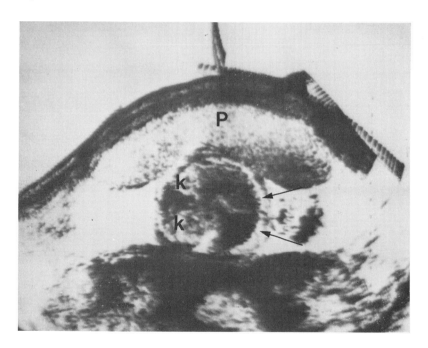

Figure 5–11. *Transverse scan showing large placenta (P) seen in Rh disease. In addition, cross section of hydropic fetus is seen with ascitic fluid (arrows pointing to white space). Note both kidneys (k) with renal collecting systems.*

The fetal liver and stomach are normally visualized by transverse scans of the upper part of the *fetal abdomen*. In some fetuses with upper intestinal obstruction, a "double bubble sign" may be seen (Fig. 5–10). In these cases, an amniogram may be helpful in verifying the diagnosis.

Fetal ascites is readily visualized by sonar (Figs. 5–11 and 5–12). Moreover, the severity of ascites may be estimated by comparing the abdominal circumference of the affected fetus with that normally expected in relation to a given week of gestation. Similarly, the rate of accumulation of ascitic fluid may be calculated from the weekly increments in the abdominal girth.

Although fetal ascites is most often attributed to Rh disease, nonimmunologic ascites (often associated with multiple congenital anomalies) has also been described and can be diagnosed by ultrasound.[17]

Garrett et al. first described the diagnosis of *polycystic kidney* at 31 weeks' gestation.[18] This author has seen two cases of multicystic kidneys (Fig. 5–13).

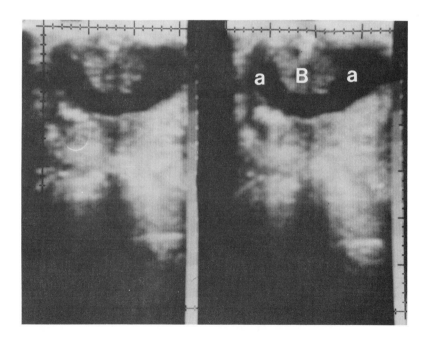

Figure 5–12.   *Cross section of fetal abdomen by real-time imaging. Note marked ascites (a). Bowel (B) in center of abdomen.*

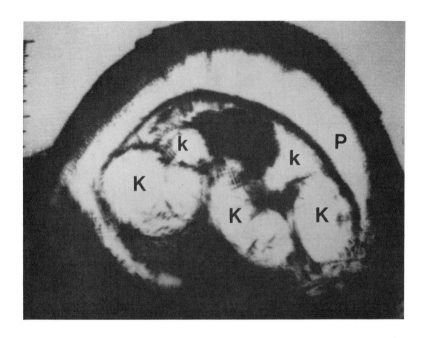

Figure 5–13. *Cross section of fetal abdomen distended with multicystic kidneys (K). Note polyhydramnios (P).*

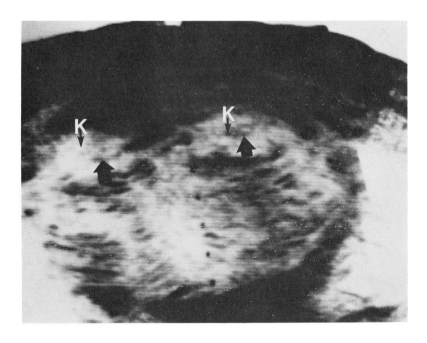

Figure 5–14. *Cross section of fetal abdomen showing kidney (K & arrow) and renal collecting systems (large arrows).*

The antenatal sonar diagnosis of *renal agenesis* may be difficult because in the absence of the kidneys, the renal tissue space is usually still preserved. Thus, to rule out renal agenesis, the renal collecting system (Fig. 5–14) and the fetal bladder (Fig. 5–15) should be clearly visualized.

Pelvic Masses. A frequent question during pregnancy is whether a palpable *pelvic mass* is uterine or ovarian in origin. Additionally, the size of some pelvic masses may be difficult to assess because of the gravid uterus. It is important to resolve these clinical problems because a large ovarian tumor may have to be surgically excised (incidence of malignancy is 2%–5%), whereas myomas during pregnancy are usually left alone.[19,20]

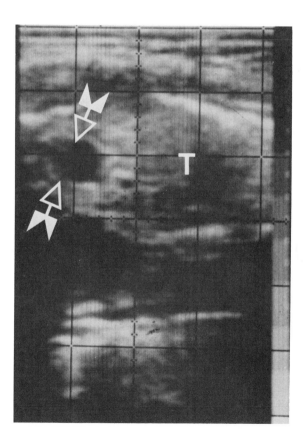

Figure 5–15. *Longitudinal scan by real-time imaging. Note fetal bladder (arrows) at lower aspect of trunk (T).*

In a large series of pregnant women, Bezjian found that he could distinguish ovarian tumors from myomas sonographically with an accuracy approaching 95%.[21] This author's experience is also similar. The difficulty usually arises when: (1) a large dense mass is seen in the cul-de-sac and a clear interface is noted between the mass and the uterus. Although more often than not, such masses are ovarian in origin, a pedunculated myoma (not common in the cul-de-sac) cannot be ruled out (Fig. 5–16). (2) A very homogeneous degenerated cystic myoma in the fundal area may resemble a cyst. In such cases, an irregular uterine outline is the only clue that may lead the sonographer to the correct diagnosis of leiomyomata.

In the majority of cases, myomas are readily recognized during pregnancy because their echo pattern at some plane not only resembles, but also merges with that of the uterus; further, the latter is enlarged and irregular in shape (Figs. 5–17 to 5–19). By contrast, in the presence of an adnexal mass, a clear demarcation (interface) between

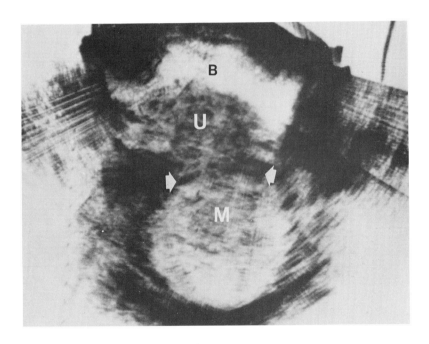

Figure 5–16. *Transverse scan of lower uterine area (U) showing an 8 × 8 cm dense mass (M) in cul-de-sac with a clear line of separation (arrows) from the uterus. This mass was explored and found to be a dermoid. However, a pedunculated myoma cannot be ruled out. B = bladder.*

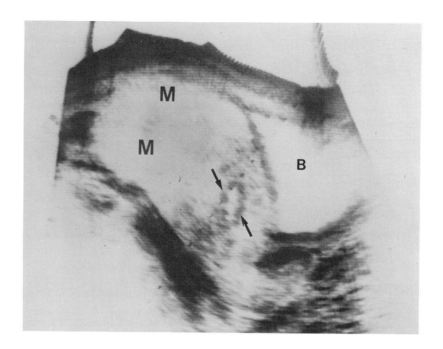

Figure 5–17. *Longitudinal scan of enlarged uterus due to myomas (M). Note the uniform echo pattern all through. A 6-week gestational sac is seen (arrows). B = bladder.*

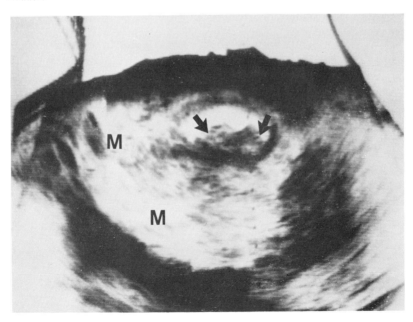

Figure 5–18. *Transverse scan of large irregular uterus. Note uniform echo pattern between myoma (M) and uterine area surrounding gestational sac. A fetus is seen (arrows) with a crown-rump length of 2.9 cm equivalent to 10⁻ weeks' gestation.*

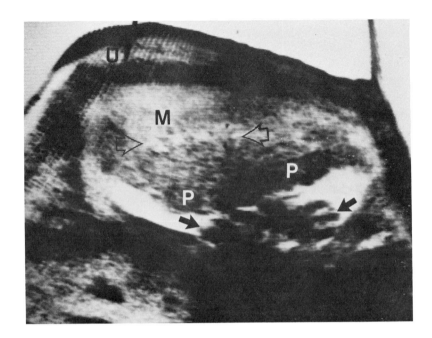

Figure 5–19. *Longitudinal scan of large uterus reaching umbilicus. Fetal crown-rump length (arrows) is only 7.2 cm, equivalent to 13 + weeks' gestation. The placenta (P) is seen overlying a myoma (M). Open arrows indicate line of demarcation between placenta and myoma.*

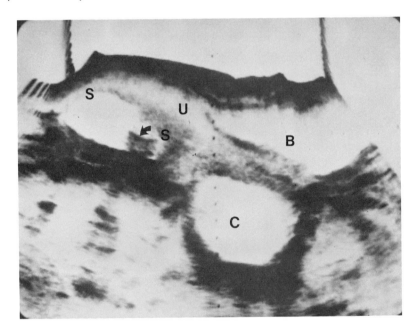

Figure 5–20. *Longitudinal scan showing a large cul-de-sac cystic ovarian mass (C) displacing a normally shaped gravid uterus. A small 8-week fetus is seen (arrow) in gestational sac (S).*

cyst and uterus is almost always present and the uterus appears regular in shape and contour (Fig. 5–20).

The obstetrician who sends a gravida suspected of having a pelvic mass to ultrasound is in a position not only to confirm his clinical impression, but also to learn about: (1) the normalcy of the pregnancy; (2) gestational age; (3) placental position (important if amniocentesis is entertained); (4) origin of the mass (uterine or adnexal); (5) nature of the mass, i.e., cystic or solid—if solid, the physician should not expect to obtain a list of the differential diagnosis of possible ovarian tumors because the echo patterns of different ovarian neoplasms are not characteristic—and (6) size of the mass.

References

1. Sabbagha, R. E., and Depp, R.: Sonar: A tool for the detection of fetal congenital anomalies. Clin. Obstet. Gynecol., 20:279, 1977.
2. Abdulla, U. et al.: Effect of diagnostic ultrasound on maternal and fetal chromosomes. Lancet, 2:829, 1971.
3. Abdulla, U. et al.: Effect of ultrasound on chromosomes of lymphocyte cultures. Br. Med. J., 3:797, 1972.
4. Bobrow, M., Blackwell, N., and Uhrau, A.: Absence of any observed effect of ultrasonic irradiation on human chromosomes. J. Obstet. Gynaecol. Br. Commonw., 78:730, 1971.
5. Boyde, E. et al.: Chromosome breakage and ultrasound. Br. Med. J., 2:501, 1971.
6. Hellman, L.M., Duffus, G.M., Donald, I., and Sunden, B.: Safety of diagnostic ultrasound in obstetrics. Lancet, 1:1133, 1970.
7. Donald, I., Morley, P., and Barnett, E.: The diagnosis of blighted ovum by sonar. J. Obstet. Gynaecol. Br. Commonw., 79:304, 1972.
8. Robinson, H. P.: The diagnosis of early pregnancy failure by sonar. Br. J. Obstet. Gynaecol., 11:849, 1975.
9. Cadkin, A. V., and Sabbagha, R. E.: Ultrasonic diagnosis of abnormal pregnancy. Clin. Obstet. Gynecol., 20:265, 1977.
10. Duff, G. B.: Prognosis in threatened abortion: A comparison between predictions made by sonar, urinary hormone assays and clinical judgement. Br. J. Obstet. Gynaecol., 82:858, 1975.
11. Jouppila, P., Piiroinen, O.: Ultrasonic diagnosis of fetal life in early pregnancy. Obstet. Gynecol., 46:616, 1975.
12. Varma, T. R.: The value of ultrasonic B-scanning in diagnosis when bleeding is present in early pregnancy. Am. J. Obstet. Gynecol., 114:607, 1972.
13. Dewhurst, C. J., Beazley, J. M., and Campbell, S.: Assessment of the fetal maturity and dysmaturity. Am. J. Obstet. Gynecol., 11e:141, 1972.
14. Campbell, S.: The assessment of fetal development by diagnostic ultrasound. Clin. Perinatol., 1:507, 1974.
15. Campbell, S.: Early prenatal diagnosis of neural tube defects by ultrasound. Clin. Obstet. Gynecol., 20:351, 1977.

16. Sabbagha, R. E., Depp, R., Grasse, D., Kipper, I.: Ultrasound diagnosis of occipitothoracic meningocele at 22 weeks' gestation. Am. J. Obstet. Gynecol., *131*:113, 1978.
17. Turski, D. M., Shahidi, N., Viseskul, C., and Gilbert, E.: Nonimmunologic hydrops fetalis. Am. J. Obstet. Gynecol., *131*:586, 1978.
18. Garrett, W. J., Grunwald, G., and Robinson, D. E.: Prenatal diagnosis of fetal polycystic kidney by ultrasound. Aust. N.Z. J. Obstet. Gynecol., *10*:7, 1970.
19. Barber, H. R.: Diagnosing and managing the unilateral mass. Contemp. Ob–Gyn, 7:99, 1976.
20. Bezjian, A. A., Caretero, M. M.: Ultrasonic evaluation of pelvic masses in pregnancy. Clin. Obstet. Gynecol., *20*:325, 1977.
21. Bezjian, A. A.: Personal communication.

6

THE PLACENTA

In a variety of antenatal conditions, it is essential for the obstetrician to learn about placental structure and position. For example, vaginal bleeding may be the first sign of some abnormality such as hydatidiform mole or placenta previa. Additionally, the placenta should be localized in women suspected of having a transverse fetal lie at term and in those seeking genetic counseling.

At present, the best method for placental localization is sonography because of its (1) speed; (2) accuracy (>95%); (3) convenience—the procedure is noninvasive and on occasion may be performed at the bedside; and (4) safety—sonar does not emit ionizing radiation.

In this chapter, the entities of hydatidiform mole, placenta previa, and abruptio are discussed. Further, the benefits of sonar examination of pregnancy prior to amniocentesis are presented.

Hydatidiform Mole

Although vaginal bleeding is sometimes associated with abnormalities of the fetus, placenta, or both (Table 6–1), in many gravidas the outcome of pregnancy may be normal. Nonetheless, early recognition of an abnormal state is extremely valuable because it permits the obstetrician to institute appropriate therapy. The diagnosis of hydatidiform mole has been markedly enhanced by sonar, and the treatment greatly simplified by suction curettage.

Table 6–1. *Etiology of Bleeding in Early Pregnancy*

Blighted ovum
Missed abortion
Hydatidiform mole
Fetal anomalies
Uterine or pelvic masses
Normal pregnancy
Other causes

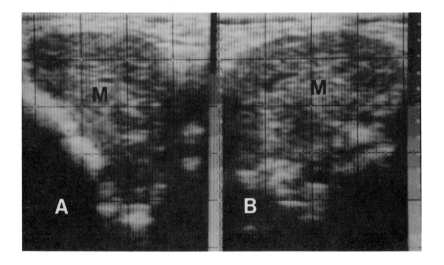

Figure 6–1. *Hydatidiform mole (M) (by real-time imaging) exhibiting classic snowstorm appearance. A, longitudinal scan with empty bladder; B, transverse scan.*

Diagnosis. The sonographic characteristics of mole are described in a number of reports.[1-4] Most investigators emphasize the so-called classic sonogram in which the uterus reflects a diffuse pattern of echoes resembling a snowstorm or snowflake appearance (Figs. 6–1 and 6–2). Characteristically, these echoes disappear at a low-gain setting (similar to echoes of normal placenta).

A number of molar placentas, however, do not exhibit the classic appearance described. The differential diagnosis of echograms resembling mole is listed in Table 6–2 and merits further discussion.

Missed Abortion Vs. Mole. In a large study, Vassilakos et al. classified molar pregnancy into two pathologic entities: partial and complete

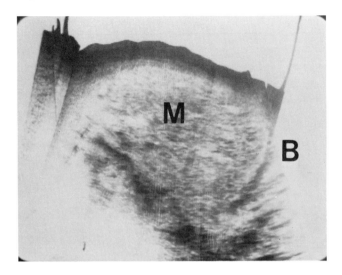

Figure 6–2. *Longitudinal scan of hydatidiform mole (M) (by gray-scale imaging) exhibiting classic snowstorm appearance. B = bladder.*

Table 6–2. *Differential Diagnosis of Echograms Resembling Hydatidiform Mole and Data Helpful in Making the Diagnosis*

Missed abortion (6–11 weeks' gestation)	Echogram is typical of mole only in "complete moles"
Intrauterine fetal death (IUFD) (12–16 weeks' gestation)	Fundal height receding. UCG* turns negative
Myoma with pregnancy	Placenta normal (i.e., compact with chorionic plate)
Without pregnancy	UCG* negative
Ovarian tumor (granulosa cell or teratoma)	
With pregnancy	Placenta normal (i.e., compact with chorionic plate)
Without pregnancy	UCG* may be positive in teratocarcinoma but uterus can be identified and shows no evidence of pregnancy
Twin gestation (10–14 weeks')	Careful search to show twins—possible by real-time imaging

*UCG—Urinary chorionic gonadotropin.

Table 6–3.   *Difference Between Partial and Complete Hydatidiform Moles*

Partial	Complete
75% of moles	25% of moles
Villi—small (0.5–5 mm) in early pregnancy	Villi—large (up to 9 cm) in early pregnancy
Usually associated with stunted fetus. Rarely, fetus remains alive until mid or late pregnancy	No fetal tissue found
Karyotype with chromosomal anomalies (trisomy, tetraploidy)	Karyotype exclusively 46 XX normal female
Rarely progresses to choriocarcinoma	2.5% progress to choriocarcinoma

(Table 6–3).[5] *Partial moles* cannot be differentiated from missed abortion in early pregnancy because the villi are small and their echo pattern is not characteristic. In addition, a gestational sac is often seen in both entities. Similarly, a stunted fetus may be readily recognized within the sac in both conditions. Because of fetal demise or absence of fetus, the pregnancy is usually terminated by the obstetrician. However, on occasion, molar tissue is discovered by the pathologist upon microscopic examination of the placenta at a later date. In contrast, *complete moles*, which are less frequent (only 25% of moles), can be differentiated from missed abortion because the villi attain a large size early in the first trimester of pregnancy.

Intrauterine Fetal Death Vs. Mole. In some moles cystic areas of varying size may be visualized. These are attributed to the presence of blood clots within molar tissue. Sometimes, interfaces between some of these clots reflect an echo pattern resembling that of a fetus (Fig. 6–3), albeit a nonliving one. Echograms of such pregnancies are most difficult to distinguish from those in which intrauterine fetal death has occurred early in the second trimester of pregnancy. Fortunately, the treatment of choice in either of these conditions is termination of pregnancy.

Pelvic Mass Vs. Mole. On occasion, the echogenic patterns of large myomas and ovarian tumors (Table 6–2) are similar to that of mole (Fig. 6–4). When associated with pregnancy, these tumors are distinguished from mole because a normal placenta (compact villi and clear chorionic plate) is visualized. In the absence of pregnancy, ovarian tumor is differentiated from mole when a normal uterus is seen songraphically.

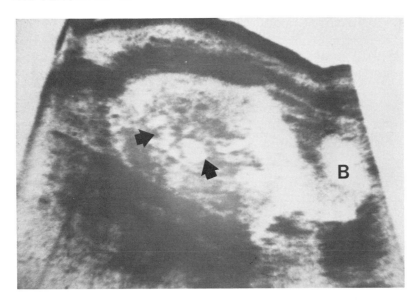

Figure 6–3. *Longitudinal scan of hydatidiform mole with large blood clots resembling dead fetus (arrows). B = bladder.*

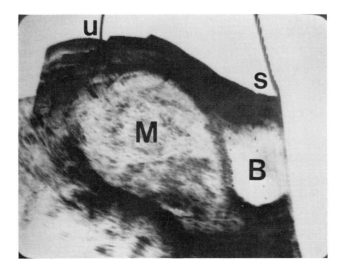

Figure 6–4. *Longitudinal scan of large myomatous uterus (M) resembling mole. B = bladder; s = symphysis pubis; u = umbilicus.*

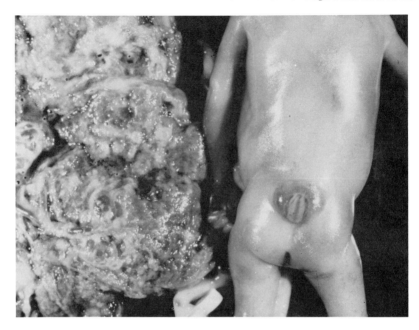

Figure 6–5.   *Second trimester fetus associated with hydatidiform mole. Note spina bifida.*

In the majority of cases of mole, careful examination by an experienced sonographer and correlation between clinical, laboratory, and sonar findings should lead to the correct diagnosis. If the ultrasound specialist is still in doubt, sonar evaluation should be repeated in about two weeks.

Mole and Fetus. Rarely, hydatidiform mole is seen in conjunction with a live fetus during the second or even third trimester of pregnancy.[6–8] The author diagnosed two such cases by ultrasound (at approximately 15 weeks' gestation), and spina bifida was noted in each fetus (Fig. 6–5). At present, sonography seems to be the only method by which this entity can be diagnosed antenatally because the fetus is not visualized radiographically (bone calcification is absent) and placental detail is not outlined by amniography. Evacuation of molar tissue by suction curettage is now possible regardless of uterine size; however, this is inadvisable in the presence of hydatidiform mole and a large fetus (beyond 12 weeks' gestation) because the procedure may be prolonged and bleeding excessive. In some gravidas and in the absence of hypertension, prostaglandin E_2 suppositories may be successfully used to induce labor and to evacuate the uterus. In others for whom prostaglandins are contraindicated and the vaginal route of delivery fails, hysterotomy or even hysterectomy may be indicated.

Placenta Previa

Ultrasound has enabled us to view the placenta as a dynamic rather than, as previously thought, a static organ.[9-10] Placental size can vary considerably in different pregnancies. For example, in certain cases of growth retardation, placental size is small whereas in gravidas who have diabetes mellitus or are sensitized by Rh antigen, placental volume is large. In the latter two conditions, it is tempting to consider excessive placental size as a response, at least in part, to a rapidly growing fetus in the presence of maternal diabetes and to fetal anemia in Rh disease.[11] Additionally, the placenta is capable, in some cases, of changing its site of implantation with advancing gestation.[12-16] As a result, a certain number of placentas visualized in a low-lying position by mid pregnancy eventually assume normal implantation, thus the name peripatetic placenta.[17]

Peripatetic Placenta. The phenomenon of ascension of a segment of the placenta from the lower uterine area in mid pregnancy to a normal position by term was first described by King[12] and verified later by others.[13-17]

In essence, it is now apparent that the placenta of mid pregnancy is a large organ covering the entire length of the uterine wall,[11] and in many gravidas it is seen extending well into the lower aspect of the uterus and covering the cervix. This placental extension should be viewed as a normal finding because the majority of these women neither bleed vaginally nor develop placenta previa at term. Despite the clarity of this relatively recent discovery, many physicians still refer to a low-lying placenta during the second trimester of pregnancy as placenta previa. It should be emphasized that placenta previa refers to a clinical diagnosis applicable to late pregnancy,[18] and its use to describe a normal second trimester entity of low placental implantation is incorrect and misleading.

The mechanism by which a positional change is effected in these low-lying placentas is difficult to understand. What is even harder to comprehend is why a small proportion of such placentas do become previas at term. Young recently detailed the mechanism that may be responsible for placental ascension.[17] He noted, first, that the basic tissue forming the placenta has the ability to reshape itself by differential growth at the cellular level—chorion frondosum multiplies and thickens whereas chorion laeve atrophies; second, he observed that the uterine fundus grows at a much faster rate than the placenta in the third trimester of pregnancy, generating a force that tends to drag and favor growth of the placenta toward the fundus. Finally, a change in the relative position of the placenta occurs by term as the lower uterine segment is developed.

It is interesting to note that Buttery and Davison, using time-lapse echography, clearly showed that Braxton-Hicks contractions (physiologic contractions followed by relaxation) occur in mid pregnancy.[18] These contractions (while they last) result in two sonographic echo patterns: (1) Anterior placentas may be displaced to the lower uterine area and appear (temporarily) to be covering the os (Figs. 6–6 and 6–7). (2) A myoma-like thickening of the posterior wall of the uterus is seen (Fig. 6–7) and disappears within minutes. These intriguing changes in the relationship of the uterus to its contents (verified by the

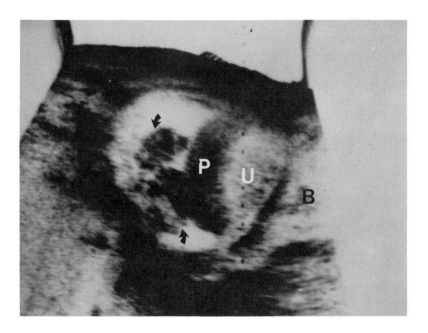

Figure 6–6. *Longitudinal scan showing placenta (P) covering lower uterine area (U). Fetus (arrows) is in a "standing" position. B = bladder area.*

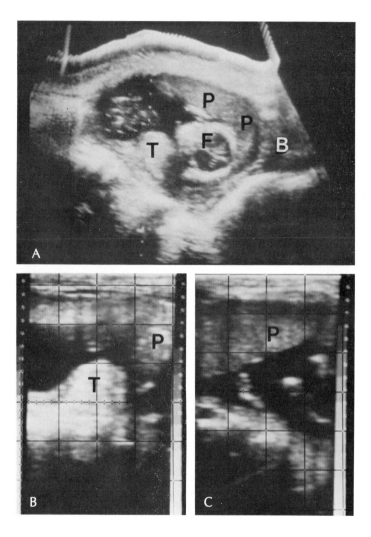

Figure 6–7. *A, Longitudinal scan at 16 weeks' gestation during Braxton-Hicks contraction. Note: (1) myoma-like thickening of posterior uterine wall (T) and its projection into uterine cavity; (2) portion of placenta (P) located anteriorly is displaced toward lower uterine area. B, Longitudinal scan obtained by real-time imaging at 16 weeks' gestation showing myoma-like projection (T) into uterine cavity and a portion of placenta (P) in lower uterine area. C, Same patient as in B scanned 5 minutes later. Uterus is relaxed. Myoma-like projection seen in B has disappeared and the placenta is no longer displaced toward the lower uterine area. B = bladder; F = fetal body.*

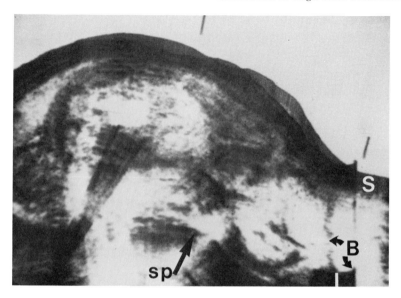

Figure 6–8. *Longitudinal scan of term pregnancy showing fetal head in pelvis. A line joining the sacral promontory (sp) to the symphysis pubis (S) demarcates the lower uterine area. The internal os of the cervix (I) is just posterior to the angle joining the base and superior wall (arrows) of the bladder (B).*

author) may explain, at least in part, the preponderance of low-lying placentas (particularly those in anterior locations) in mid pregnancy.

Diagnosis of Placenta Previa. Placental position should be ascertained by ultrasound in gravidas who present with vaginal bleeding or a transverse lie at term.[16] The diagnosis of placenta previa depends on evaluating the position of the placenta in relation to the lower uterine segment and to the internal os of the cervix.

Anatomic Landmarks. The lower uterine segment is clearly identifiable on echograms as the area below a line that joins the symphysis pubis to the sacral promontory (Fig. 6–8).[11] The internal os of the cervix is posterior to the junction of the base and superior wall of the

Figure 6–9. *Longitudinal scans of same gravida with different degrees of bladder (B) filling. As the bladder is filled: The base (arrow) moves posteriorly and the superior wall (arrow) becomes slightly convex and then concave; and the angle of junction between base and superior wall of bladder is displaced posteriorly but does not alter location of internal os of cervix (I). Note relative change of placenta (P) when bladder is minimally distended (A) and markedly distended (C).*

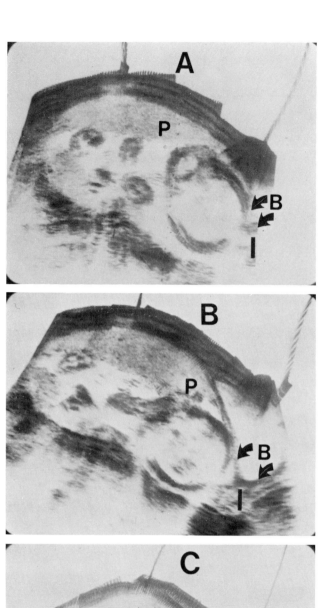

bladder[20] (Figure 6–8)—an angle relatively constant in position if bladder distention is moderate. In scanning pregnant women to rule out placenta previa, an overly distended bladder should be absolutely avoided because it may displace an anteriorly or posteriorly located placenta toward the cervix.[21] As a result, the sonographer may make a false diagnosis of placenta previa. In fact, in one large study, false positive diagnoses of placenta previa were clearly attributed to an overfilled bladder (Fig. 6–9).[22] Gottesfeld recommends postvoid sonographic evaluation of placental position prior to making the diagnosis of placenta previa.[23]

If placental echoes are visualized in the lower uterine segment by the latter part of the third trimester of pregnancy, the diagnosis of a low-lying placenta previa is made. If, on the other hand, placental echoes are seen encroaching upon the cervical area, the diagnosis of either partial or total previa is made—depending upon the extent to which the cervix is covered. Sometimes the distinction between partial and total placenta previa may be difficult. However, in the presence of

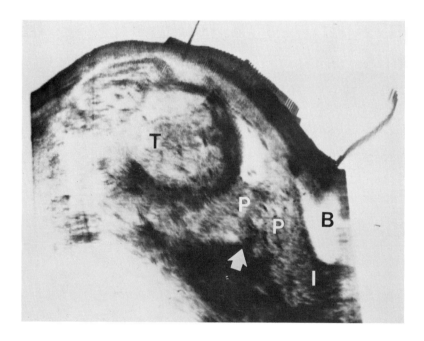

Figure 6–10. *Longitudinal scan showing complete posterior placenta previa (PP) and fetal trunk (T) displaced out of the pelvis. B = bladder; I = internal os of cervix; arrow pointing to sacral promontory.*

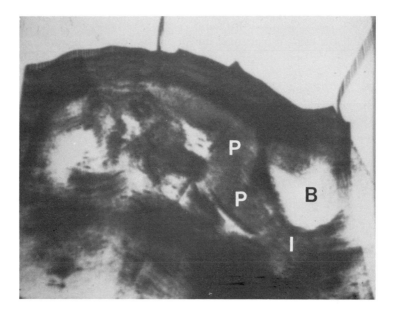

Figure 6–11. *Longitudinal scan of anterior complete placenta previa (P). Note fetus completely displaced out of pelvis. B = bladder; I = internal os of cervix.*

a frank previa, the presenting part is usually at some distance from either the superior wall of the bladder or the sacral promontory (at least 15 mm from the upper part of the sacrum) (Figs. 6–10 and 6–11).[12]

Differential Diagnosis. In the majority of pregnancies, placenta previa can be excluded with absolute certainty by ultrasound. Such exclusion may also be performed in the labor suite using small portable real-time equipment. In the absence of placenta previa, vaginal bleeding is usually attributed to placental abruption, and vaginal examination for assessment of cervical dilatation, station, presenting part, and fetal status (by electronic fetal monitoring with scalp electrode) may be permissible without a double set-up examination. Nonetheless, it should be emphasized that the lower edge of the placenta, particularly if implantation is along the lateral uterine wall, may on occasion be difficult to assess sonographically. Similarly, in some patients the distinction between a low-lying placenta and placenta previa may be difficult, particularly when using real-time imaging. Under these circumstances, the ultrasound report should be clearly descriptive of the findings and the patient managed in accordance with established clinical principles.

In the usual case of placental abruption the sonographic appearance of the placenta is normal. However, on occasion, a retroplacental clot, if present, is visible by ultrasound and resembles echo-free choriodecidual sinuses seen in mature placentas, usually after 28 weeks' gestation.[24]

Ultrasound in Amniocentesis

Amniocentesis is an integral part of modern obstetrics. Its use extends to three general areas:

1. *Genetic studies.* Genetic counseling is recommended for gravidas at high risk of giving birth to offspring with: (a) chromosomal abnormalities, e.g., risk is 1/100 if maternal age is 40 to 44 years; (b) certain specific mendelian disorders—risk is calculated in relation to nature of disorder and to gene involved (generally 25% if recessive and 50% if dominant); and (c) congenital anomalies attributed to a multifactorial (polygenic) mode of inheritance—recurrence risk is 2% to 5%.

The amniotic fluid withdrawn is analyzed for α-fetoprotein[26] or cultured for evaluation of: chromosomal number and structure; definition of fetal sex; and measurement of specific enzyme activity or product (60–80 of 1200 enzyme deficiency diseases can be diagnosed in utero).

2. *Evaluation of fetal status.* The level of some amniotic fluid components is used to reflect fetal status. For example: the Δ OD 450 of the bilirubin-like pigment in amniotic fluid is used to evaluate the severity of Rh sensitization; the creatinine value, if greater than 2 mg%, may indicate attainment of fetal maturity; and the lecithin to sphingomyelin ratio is widely accepted as an index of fetal pulmonary maturity.[27–29]

3. *Pregnancy termination.* Intra-amniotic instillation of abortifacient agents is used to induce termination of second trimester pregnancies.

Complications of Amniocentesis. The procedure of amniocentesis is associated with a small risk, estimated at 0.5%, of complications such as: infection, hemorrhage, leakage of amniotic fluid, precipitated abortion, fetal injury, serious fetal bleed, and Rh immunization.[30,31] Additionally, contamination of amniotic fluid with blood (incidence 5–10%) may alter the assay for surfactant,[32] invalidate α-fetoprotein determinations,[33] and render interpretation of bilirubin content difficult.[29]

Attempts to enter the amniotic cavity "blindly," i.e., without evaluation of the pregnancy by ultrasound, may increase the incidence of complications and frequency of bloody taps cited above. Consequently, the routine use of ultrasound prior to amniocentesis performed for genetic studies has been recommended by the American College of Obstetricians and Gynecologists.[31]

A number of studies support this recommendation. Miskin et al.,[34] Harrison et al.,[35] and Kerenyi and Walker[38] reported a 10,- 3,- and 2-fold decrease in the incidence of bloody taps, respectively, when the placenta was localized by ultrasound prior to amniocentesis.

In contrast, other studies do not demonstrate a decrease in the incidence of bloody taps by using sonography prior to amniocentesis.[37–39]

For various reasons, it is difficult to compare all these studies or even draw definite conclusions from any one of them.

1. The *skill* and *experience* of both the sonographer and the physician drawing amniotic fluid have not been carefully weighed and analyzed; these factors are apt to influence markedly the success with which clear amniotic fluid is withdrawn.

2. The *degree of bladder filling* has not been defined. It is now known that the accuracy of placenta localization is related to the degree of bladder distention, particularly during the second trimester of pregnancy.[21] An overly distended bladder may displace the lower part of the uterus and change the relationship between the placenta and the uterine wall.[22] After the 12th week of gestation, visualization of the contents of the uterus is possible with a minimally distended bladder.

3. The *interval* between the ultrasound examination and amniocentesis is not uniform—it is best to draw amniotic fluid in the ultrasound room or at least adjacent to it and soon after the completion of sonography.

4. Definition of what constitutes a *"bloody tap"* is not standardized. In some studies, if the fluid sample first withdrawn contained blood, but cleared immediately, the "tap" was not considered bloody, and the initial contamination was attributed to blood from the abdominal wall or myometrium. In other studies, a "tap" was considered bloody if at any time the fluid did not appear to be clear.

5. Techniques are not standardized, e.g., needle gauge.

The author believes that the benefits of ultrasonic evaluation of pregnancy prior to amniocentesis outweigh any potential and as yet unidentified risks of sonar. These benefits extend beyond reduction in the incidence of maternal and fetal complications or even the frequency of bloody taps already discussed and include: (1) prevention of fetal-maternal transfusion and possible immunization of Rh-negative gravidas—achieved by delineation of a window or site for entry into the amniotic sac without penetrating the placenta;[35, 39-42] (2) determination of fetal age (see Chap. 3) to ensure that amniocentesis is performed at the most optimal time for successful withdrawal of amniotic fluid, i.e., approximately 16 weeks' gestation; (3) detection of multiple pregnancy and withdrawal of amniotic fluid from areas within each sac; (4) detection of leiomyomata or adnexal masses previously unnoticed. In the presence of myomas, amniocentesis is much more likely to be successful following ultrasonic localization of a "pocket" of amniotic fluid. In the presence of an ovarian mass, careful follow-up of the pregnancy is mandatory; and (5) discovery of congenital anomalies.

Technique of Amniocentesis. In the author's laboratory, the following steps are adhered to prior to amniocentesis. First, the gravida is scanned with a completely empty bladder. In this way placental position is neither distorted by the bladder nor altered when the patient is asked to empty her bladder prior to amniocentesis.

Second, the physician doing the "tap" is physically present in the sonar room and watches the scan as it is performed. As a result, he formulates a mental image of the relationship between fetal lie, placental position, and direction of the needle to be used for amniocentesis.

Although in approximately 50% of gravidas the placenta is located in an anterior position and is seen along a midline plane (between umbilicus and symphysis pubis) (Fig. 6–12), its main body, in the majority of cases, actually covers either the right or left side of the anterior uterine wall. As a result, amniocentesis may be performed on the opposite side.

In the author's laboratory, the suprapubic location (either midline or 1–2 cm to either side) is the site most frequently chosen for amniocentesis; at this location, the tip of the needle is angled cephalad so that it penetrates the uterine wall perpendicularly. Occasionally, however, amniocentesis is done through the uterine fundus (Fig. 6–12).

Biopsy Transducers. Goldberg and Pollack[44] and Bang and Northeved[45] devised an ultrasound transducer with a central aperture of sufficient width to allow insertion of an aspiration-biopsy needle.

The echoes produced by an aspiration ultrasonic transducer are processed to an A-mode read-out.[46] An acoustic interface is created when the tip of the needle reaches a fluid compartment and the echo is recorded as a vertical deflection of the time-base sweep.[47]

Aspiration transducers may be used to monitor removal of fluid from cysts or within various compartments of the body such as thorax,

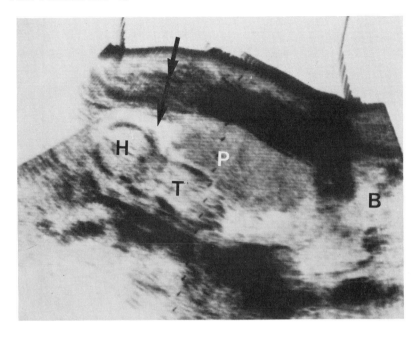

Figure 6–12.   *Longitudinal scan showing large anterior placenta (P). A transverse scan showed the placenta to be situated more to the right side. Amniocentesis may be done either in left lower quadrant or fundally (arrow).*

pericardium and abdomen. Additionally, these transducers have been used for suprapubic aspiration of urine for bacteriologic examination[48] and for amniocentesis.

In our laboratory, amniocentesis is done through an area of the maternal abdomen located by B-scan or real-time imaging. The aspiration transducer is not used routinely, for three reasons: (1) Satisfactory results are obtained by two-dimensional imaging. (2) An aspiration transducer has to be carefully sterilized; Donald has some doubts about asepsis in the central lumen of such transducers.[49] (3) Its use can be time consuming and involve the assistance of two technologists.

References

1. MacVicar, J., and Donald, I.: Sonar in the diagnosis of early pregnancy and its complications. J. Obstet. Gynaecol. Br. Commonw., *70*:387–395, 1963.
2. Gottesfeld, K. R., Taylor, E. S., Thompson, H. E., et al.: Diagnosis of hydatidiform mole by ultrasound. Obstet. Gynecol., *30*:163–171, 1967.

3. Kohorn, E. I., Morrison, J., Ashford, C., et al.: Ultrasonic scanning in obstetrics and gynecology. Obstet. Gynecol., *34*:515–522, 1969.
4. Leopold, G. R.: Diagnostic ultrasound in the detection of molar pregnancy. Radiology, *98*:171–176, 1971.
5. Vassilakos, P., Riotton, G., Tadashi, K.: Hydatidiform mole: two entities. Am. J. Obstet. Gynecol., *127*:167, 1977.
6. Ballas, S., Peyser, M. R., and Toaff, R.: Diagnosis of hydatidiform mole with and without coexistent fetus by nonstored image echography. Obstet. Gynecol., *50*:182, 1977.
7. Hohe, P. T., Cochrane, C. R., Gmelich, J. T., and Austin, J. A.: Coexistent trophoblastic tumor and viable pregnancy. Obstet. Gynecol., *38*:899, 1971.
8. Szulman, A. E., and Surti, U.: The syndromes of hydatidiform mole; I. Cytogenetic and morphologic correlations. Am. J. Obstet. Gynecol., *131*:665, 1978.
9. Crawford, J. M.: A study of human placental growth with observations on the placenta in erythroblastosis foetalis. J. Obstet. Gynaecol. Br. Commonw., *66*:885, 1959.
10. Wynn, R. M.: Principles of placentation and early human placental development. *In* The Placenta. Edited by P. Gruenwald. Lancaster Medical and Technical Publishing Co., Ltd., 1975.
11. Sabbagha, R. E.: Ultrasound in managing the high-risk pregnancy. *In* Management of the High-Risk Pregnancy. Edited by W. N. Spellacy. Baltimore, University Park Press, 1976.
12. King, D. L.: Placental migration demonstrated by ultrasonography. A hypothesis of dynamic placentation. Radiology, *109*:167–170, 1973.
13. Young, G. B.: The ascending placenta—an analysis of 230 placental arteriograms, 1964–1974. Abstracts of 3rd Congress of European Association of Radiology, Edinburgh. Abstract No. 254, 1975.
14. Badria, L., and Young, G. B.: Correlation of ultrasonic and soft tissue x-ray placentography in 300 cases. J. Clin. Ultrasound, *4*:403–407, 1976.
15. Bell, R. L.: Placental migration. J. Tenn. Med. Assoc., *69*:341, 1976.
16. Edelstone, D. I.: Placental localization by ultrasound. Clin. Obstet. Gynecol., *20*:285, 1977.
17. Young, G. B.: The peripatetic placenta. Radiology, *128*:183–188, 1978.
18. Buttery, B. and Davison, G.: The dynamic uterus revealed by time-lapse echography. J. Clin. Ultrasound, *6*:19–22, 1978.
19. Robertson, J. G.: Placenta praevia. Practitioner, *204*:383–392, 1970.
20. Gray, H., Gray's Anatomy. Edited by P. T. Pick, and R. Howden. New York, Bounty Books, 1977.
21. Zemlyn, S.: The effect of the urinary bladder in obstetrical sonography. Radiology, *128*:169, 1978.
22. Bowie, J. D., Rochester, D., Cadkin, A. V., Cooke, W. T., and Kunzmann, A.: Accuracy of placental localization by ultrasound. Radiology, *128*:177–180, 1978.
23. Gottesfeld, K. R.: Ultrasound in obstetrics. Clin. Obstet. Gynecol., *21*:311, 1978.
24. Fisher, C. C., Garrett, W., and Kossoff, G.: Placental aging monitored by gray scale echography. Am. J. Obstet. Gynecol., *124*:483, 1976.
25. Thompson, M. W.: Counseling in genetics and cytogenetics. *In* Perinatal Medicine. Edited by J. Goodwin, J. Godden, and G. Chance. Baltimore, Williams & Wilkins Co., 1976.
26. Cowchock, F. S.: Use of alpha-feto protein in prenatal diagnosis. Clin. Obstet. Gynecol., *19*:871, 1976.

27. Liley, A. W.: Errors in the assessment of hemolytic disease from amniotic fluid. Am. J. Obstet. Gynecol., 86:485, 1963.
28. Pitkin, R. M.: Fetal maturity: Nonlipid amniotic fluid assessment. In Management of the High-Risk Pregnancy. Edited by W. N. Spellacy. Baltimore, University Park Press, 1976.
29. Gluck, L.: Fetal maturity and amniotic fluid surfactant determinations. In Management of the High-Risk Pregnancy. Edited by W. N. Spellacy. Baltimore, University Park Press, 1976.
30. NICHD National Registry for Amniocentesis Study Group: Midtrimester amniocentesis for prenatal diagnosis. Safety and accuracy. J.A.M.A., 236:1471, 1976.
31. Schwarz, R. H., and Mennuti, M. T.: Antenatal diagnosis of genetic disorders. Am. Coll. Obstet. Gynecol., Tech. Bulletin 39, 1976.
32. Buhl, W. C., and Spellacy, W. N.: Effects of blood or meconium on the determination of the amniotic fluid lecithin/sphingomyelin ratio. Am. J. Obstet. Gynecol., 121:321, 1975.
33. Doran, T. A. et al.: The antenatal diagnosis of genetic disease. Am. J. Obstet. Gynecol., 118:314, 1974.
34. Miskin, M. et al.: Use of ultrasound for placental localization in genetic amniocentesis. Obstet. Gynecol., 43:872, 1974.
35. Harrison, R., Campbell, S., and Craft, I.: Risks of fetomaternal hemorrhage resulting from amniocentesis with and without ultrasound placental localization. Obstet. Gynecol., 46:389, 1975.
36. Kerenyi, T. D., and Walker, B.: The preventability of "bloody taps" in second trimester amniocentesis by ultrasound scanning. Obstet. Gynecol., 50:61, 1977.
37. Gerbie, A. B., and Shkolnik, A. A.: Ultrasound prior to amniocentesis for genetic counseling. Obstet. Gynecol., 46:716, 1975.
38. Karp, L. E. et al.: Ultrasonic placental localization and bloody taps in midtrimester amniocentesis for prenatal diagnosis. Obstet. Gynecol., 50:589, 1977.
39. Young, P. E., Matson, M. R., and Jones, O. W.: Amniocentesis for prenatal diagnosis. Review of problems and outcomes in a large series. Am. J. Obstet. Gynecol., 125:495, 1976.
40. Lawrence, M.: Diagnostic amniocentesis in early pregnancy. Br. Med. J., 2:191, 1977.
41. Peddle, L. J.: Increase of antibody titer following amniocentesis. Am. J. Obstet. Gynecol., 100:567, 1968.
42. Queenan, J. T., and Adams, D. W.: Amniocentesis: A possible immunizing hazard. Obstet. Gynecol., 24:530, 1964.
43. Robinson, A.: Intrauterine diagnosis and ultrasound. Lancet, 2:1504, 1973.
44. Goldberg, B. B., and Pollack, H. M.: Ultrasonic aspiration transducer. Radiology, 102:187, 1972.
45. Bang, J., and Northeved, A.: A new ultrasonic method for transabdominal amniocentesis. Am. J. Obstet. Gynecol., 114:599, 1972.
46. Goldberg, B. B., and Pollack, H. M.: Ultrasonic aspiration-biopsy transducer. Radiology, 108:667, 1973.
47. Goldberg, B. B., and Ziskin, M. C.: Echo patterns with an aspiration ultrasonic transducer. Invest. Radiol., 8:78, 1973.
48. Goldberg, B. B., and Meyer, H.: Ultrasonically guided suprapubic urinary bladder aspiration. Pediatrics, 51:70, 1973.
49. Donald, I.: Further developments in diagnostic sonar in obstetrics and gynecology. In Obstetrics and Gynecology Annual: 1977. Edited by R. M. Wynn. New York, Appleton-Century-Crofts, 1977.

INDEX

Page numbers in *italics* indicate illustrations;
page numbers followed by t indicate tables.